Surgical Infections

I dedicate this book to all my registrars who have taught me how little I really know

Surgical Infections

Alan Pollock
BSc, MB, ChB, FRCS(Eng), FRCS(Ed)

Consultant Surgeon, Scarborough Health District
Hunterian Professor, Royal College of Surgeons of England

Microbiology and Immunology
by Charles Easmon
MD, PhD, MRCPath

Professor of Medical Microbiology
St Mary's Hospital, London

with Mary Evans BA

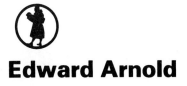

Edward Arnold

© Alan Pollock 1987

First published in Great Britain 1987 by
Edward Arnold (Publishers) Ltd, 41 Bedford Square, London WC1B 3DQ

Edward Arnold (Australia) Pty Ltd, 80 Waverley Road, Caulfield East,
Victoria 3145, Australia

Edward Arnold, 3 East Read Street, Baltimore, Maryland 21202, U.S.A.

British Library Cataloguing in Publication Data

Pollock, Alan
   Surgical infections.
   1. Surgical wound infections
   I. Title II. Easmon, C.S.F. III. Evans, Mary
   617'.01   RD98.3

   ISBN 0-7131-4500-5

Text set in 10/11 pt Compugraphic Times
by Colset Private Limited, Singapore
Printed and bound in Great Britain by
Richard Clay Ltd, Bungay, Suffolk

Preface

This is a book for practising surgeons. It is neither a compilation of research papers, nor a textbook of microbiology (although I am deeply indebted to Professor Charles Easmon for the introductory chapters on microbiology and immunology). Its purpose is to guide surgeons in the practical management of infections. It is a personal statement, and may therefore often be controversial. I have, however, given alternative or conflicting views whenever possible, while sticking to the main purpose – that it must be a practical guide.

The book is divided into five sections. The first concerns microbiology, immunology and antimicrobial drugs. The next part deals with the metabolic and haemodynamic consequences of sepsis, the sequence of organ failure, sepsis scores and intensive care units. In the third I discuss the evaluation of prophylactic and therapeutic regimens. This is followed by a section on those community-acquired infections which concern surgeons. The fifth section is on hospital-acquired infections, their recognition, prophylaxis and treatment, and the final chapter concerns infections in patients whose immunity is compromised by malnutrition, disease or therapy.

I am grateful to many friends all over the world for their constructive help and criticism, and particularly to members of the Hospital Infection Society (UK) and the Surgical Infection Society (USA).

Scarborough 1986   AVP

Contents

Part I

Microbiology and Immunology

1

Microorganisms of concern to the surgeon

Microorganisms of concern to surgeons fall into two categories: those that present an infectious risk to the surgical team and those that cause post operative infections with or without the added danger of cross infection.

Infectious risks to surgical team

Two organisms are of primary concern here: Hepatitis B virus and Human Immunodeficiency Virus (HIV) also known as Lymphadenopathy Associated Virus (LAV). Although both viruses can be found in a range of body fluids, blood is the main route of transmission.

Hepatitis B virus (HBV)

HBV attacks liver parenchyma cells. In severe cases this results in liver damage which can be fatal. Although most individuals recover completely, in some the disease becomes chronic, and is closely associated with primary carcinoma of the liver. The most dangerous for surgeons are patients who become chronic carriers and whose blood is infectious.

In hospital HBV is transmitted by cuts or needle stick injuries contaminated by infected blood. The incubation period following inoculation is long (60–100 days).

The carrier state can be detected by the presence of Hepatitis B antigen in serum. The first marker used was the surface antigen (HBsAg), formerly known as Australia antigen. Unfortunately, this does not discriminate between infectious and non-infectious carriers. Infectivity is more closely associated with the presence of e antigen (HBeAg). An individual who is HbsAg positive should be tested for both e antibody and e antigen. Table 1.1 shows the interpretation of results.

Table 1.1 Interpretation of e antigen and antibody results in an HBsAg positive individual

e	antigen positive	Infectious
e	antibody positive	Not infectious
e	antigen/antibody negative	Infectious

The main protection against hepatitis B is good surgical technique. Known infectious cases should be dealt with at the end of the list. All samples should be labelled as 'risk of infection', using the hospital's agreed biohazard symbol. Other diagnostic departments where invasive techniques are carried out (e.g. radiology and cardiac catheterization) should be warned of the risk of blood spillage. Where this occurs sodium hypochlorite or glutaraldehyde should be used as disinfectant, but hypochlorite should not be used on metal surfaces.

The carrier does not need source isolation unless he or she is bleeding or incontinent. If a member of the surgical team is thought to have been infected by contamination of a cut or by a needle stick or other 'sharps' injury, the injury should be thoroughly cleaned and the incident reported to the Staff Health Department. They will arrange for blood to be taken for HBV serology. If the individual has no pre-existing antibody, hepatitis B immune globulin is available and should be given.

A vaccine is now available, the full course costing about £70. As HBV cannot yet be grown in culture, vaccine is prepared from infected blood. At one time there was a fear that vaccine might transmit the agent associated with the Acquired Immune Deficiency Syndrome (AIDS). However, current knowledge about HIV and epidemiological follow-up of those given vaccine show that these fears were unfounded. Surgeons have not been regarded as a high priority group to receive this vaccine.

A mild form of hepatitis known as non-A non-B can also be transmitted by blood. There are no specific tests for this form of hepatitis as no agent has yet been identified. Non-A non-B hepatitis is primarily associated with blood transfusion.

HIV

This virus is transmitted by blood. Far less is known about its infectivity than about HBV, but from the few cases of sero-conversion that have occurred it seems that a relatively large injection of blood (over 100 μl) may be necessary. Virus isolation is still a research technique, and routine testing depends on the detection of HIV antibody. The current generation of antibody detection tests are based on immunoassays. These can produce both false positive and false negative results, and all positive tests need to be confirmed by a more cumbersome technique known as Western blotting or Immuno-blotting.

It is important to realize that as yet full reliance cannot be placed on laboratory tests for HIV antibody. Most individuals with antibody have no signs or symptoms. How many will develop AIDS is unknown, but HIV infection does not equal AIDS. AIDS is simply the most serious manifestation of HIV infection. Unless bleeding or incontinent, HIV positive patients do not require source isolation. It may be desirable to nurse patients with AIDS in single rooms for reasons unconnected with infection control.

Individuals at high risk of being infected with HIV are shown in Table 1.2. Now that tests are readily available for HIV antibody there is considerable debate as to whether such tests should be applied to those within the high risk groups who need surgery. Does such testing need patient's consent, given the consequences of a positive result? What if consent is requested and refused? Are the tests good enough to justify their use in this way? How far should the clinician go in determing whether a patient falls into this group? Is proper counselling available to cope with the needs of individuals found to be positive? As yet there are no clear answers to any of these questions, but surgeons should be aware that this is a complex area where decisions may not be as easy to make as might be thought.

Table 1.2 Groups at particular risk of HIV infection

Male homosexuals or bisexuals
Haemophiliacs known or suspected of having received
   contaminated blood products
Intravenous drug abusers
Individuals recently resident in Central Africa
Heterosexual partners of above groups
Babies born to infected mothers

Clinically, the evidence to date is that HIV is likely to be a lesser risk to surgeons than hepatitis B and that the virus is not particularly resistant to chemical disinfectants. Patients, and their samples, with HIV antibody should be handled on the same way as hepatitis B patients and carriers.

Organisms that present a risk to the patient

The postoperative patient is a prime target for infection. The wound, the presence of surgical prostheses, intravenous lines and drains, are all potential sites of infection. The patient may well have reduced resistance to infection following major surgery quite apart from the underlying condition and the effects of any pre-operative chemotherapy.

Infection may be **endogenous** from the patient's own bacterial flora, or **exogenous**, resulting from cross infection. Major outbreaks of surgical infection are fortunately rare; so too are infections with highly virulent organisms such as group A beta haemolytic streptococci and *Clostridium perfringens* (welchii). Most surgical sepsis is caused by staphylococci, Gram-negative bacilli and non-sporing anaerobes. The site of the surgery and the presence of foreign bodies inserted into the patient are the prime determinants of infection.

Gram-positive bacteria

The main pathogenic genera are *Staphylococcus, Streptococcus* and *Clostridium*. Less commonly, corynebacteria can cause problems.

Staphylococcus

Staphylococci are Gram-positive organisms that grow in clusters. The main differentiation is between the coagulase-positive *Staph. aureus* and the coagulase-negative *Staph. epidermidis*.

Staph. aureus is the classical staphylococcal pathogen. It is carried in the nose and on the skin in the axilla, groin and perineum. Carriage rates may exceed 30 per cent of hospital staff and are higher than in the general population. Strains of *Staph. aureus* found in hospital tend to be more resistant to antibiotics than those found in the community. After admission patients soon become colonized with the prevalent hospital strains.

Staph. aureus is an important cause of postoperative sepsis and can cause problems at any site. Where surgery involves a prosthesis, as in vascular and orthopaedic surgery, infection is particularly severe and the presence of the foreign body may prevent successful antimicrobial therapy. Intravenous lines are a common site of *Staph. aureus* sepsis and if ignored can lead to septicaemia.

The patient may be infected in theatre or the ward with his or her own staphylococci. Infection can also occur as a result of cross infection. Where an epidemic strain of *Staph. aureus* occurs, capable of rapid spread within hospital, cross infection can result in many cases within hours. Only prompt screening and isolation of infected and colonized patients and removal of affected staff from duty will control the situation, and even this may not be immediately successful.

Phage typing is used to follow outbreaks of staphylococcal infection, but this technique is not available to most diagnostic laboratories. Initial infection control will depend upon clinical information and on any characteristics of the epidemic strain that can be readily tested in the laboratory (e.g. antibiotic sensitivity pattern).

Infection control measures are inconvenient and may cause considerable disruption to operating lists. Wards and theatres may need to be closed and cleaned and staff sent off duty. It is important, however, that there is full co-operation and understanding between the infection control team and the surgical teams. The attitude of senior staff on both sides will set the tone.

Until recently *Staph. epidermidis* was not regarded as a pathogen. Unlike *Staph. aureus* it is a true skin commensal. Now, with the increased use of prostheses and intravenous lines,*Staph. epidermidis* is recognized as an increasingly important cause of postoperative local sepsis and septicaemia. It is almost invariably associated with foreign bodies such as intravenous lines, artificial heart valves and other surgical prostheses. *Staph. epidermidis* is less virulent than *Staph. aureus*, and the course of infection is slower. However, failure to recognize it as a cause of infection can result in serious, even fatal, infection. Unfortunately, hospital strains of *Staph. epidermidis* are usually more resistant to antibiotics than *Staph. aureus*.

Cross infection does not seem to be a major problem with *Staph. epidermidis*, although outbreaks of infection have occurred in cardiothoracic units.

Streptococcus

This genus is a heterogeneous group which contains a large number of species with widely differing pathogenic potential. As far as infections in surgical patients are concerned they can be divided into four main groups:

- *Strep. pneumoniae*,
- virulent beta haemolytic streptococci,
- anaerobic streptococci,
- viridans group streptococci.

Strep. pneumoniae

This is the most common cause of postoperative pneumonia. In approximately 33 per cent of patients this is associated with bacteraemia. After surgery, pneumococcal pneumonia may present a diagnostic problem, particularly when the patient has received antibiotics. It can be difficult to get a good sputum sample, and this may be overgrown with Gram-negative bacilli. Cross infection is not a problem with *Strep. pneumoniae*.

Beta haemolytic streptococci

Cross infection involving these organisms is important. Pharyngitis, skin lesions and asymptomatic nasal carriage are all potential sources of group A streptococci, the most virulent of all the beta haemolytic streptococci. Group A streptococci cause wound infections and septicaemia, and they can occur in any type of surgery. Group C and G organisms cause a similar pattern of disease, but are less virulent than group A streptococci.

Strep. milleri (group F) is the most common streptococcus isolated from abscesses. These can be localized intraperitoneally or in the liver, or may produce metastatic abscesses in the brain. When first isolated *Strep. milleri* may only grow under anaerobic conditions. It must not however, be confused with anaerobic streptococci as it is not sensitive to metronidazole. Faecal streptococci (Group D) are normal inhabitants of the gastro-intestinal tract and can cause intra-abdominal sepsis associated with gut or biliary tract surgery. They are an important cause of urinary tract infections. Sepsis at any of these sites may progress to septicaemia.

Anaerobic cocci

The true anaerobic cocci are normal inhabitants of the mouth, the gastro-intestinal tract and the female genital tract, and they are primarily associated with surgery involving these sites. They are slow growing, fastidious organisms, usually isolated with other anaerobic species and of low virulence. They are difficult to grow, and therefore the main problem is establishing a diagnosis. Good quality specimens that arrive in the laboratory quickly are essential.

'Viridans' streptococci

This is the term used to describe a group of streptococci found in the mouth, including *Strep. mutans, Strep. mitis* and *Strep. sanguis*. They can cause problems in dental surgery and surgery of the head and neck. Other than infections caused by these organisms, the only important infections are dental caries and infective endocarditis in patients with bad teeth and abnormal heart valves. Occasionally, endocarditis occurs in patients with artificial valves and valve replacement may be necessary.

Clostridium

The members of this genus are all anaerobes and form spores. Both features play an important role in most clostridial infections. Three species are important in surgical patients: *C. perfringens* (welchii), *C. tetani* and more recently, *C. difficile*.

C. perfringens is a normal inhabitant of the human gut. Spores may be found on the skin anywhere from the waist to the thigh. If pre-operative skin disinfection fails to remove these spores, they may be introduced into the wound during surgery. Clostridial spores need warmth and anaerobic conditions to germinate and multiply. Anaerobiasis may be provided by the presence of necrotic tissue, haematoma or simply poor tissue perfusion as a result of impaired blood supply. Clostridial spores are present in soil, and large wounds with dirt and foreign bodies also provide an ideal site for the growth of *C. perfringens*. Cross infection plays no part in this infection unless there is a major failure of sterilization procedures in theatre.

Patients undergoing hip replacement or above knee amputations are particularly at risk of *C. perfringens* sepsis. *C. perfringens* produces a number of toxic products, and infections can lead to intravascular haemolysis, renal failure and extensive tissue necrosis with production of gas in the tissues. Patients with deep closed wounds will already be seriously ill by the time the first local signs of gas gangrene are noticed. Treatment consists of surgical debridement to remove necrotic tissue, dirt and foreign bodies, which contribute to wound anaerobiasis, antibiotics (e.g. benzylpenicillin) to treat infection and hyperbaric oxygen.

C. tetani flourishes in wounds which are similar to those in which *C. perfringens* thrives, and the same conditions are required for germination of both organisms. It is not, however, a normal human gut commensal and *C. tetani* spores are environmental contaminants. Part of the bacteriological screening needed in operating theatres when building work has been done is aimed at the detection of *C. tetani* spores. In older buildings plasterwork may contain horse hair which is often heavily contaminated with these spores.

Tetanus toxin acts on the central nervous system to remove inhibition of neurological responses. The result is spastic paralysis. Once the toxin begins to act it cannot be reversed and the patient must be given supportive therapy until the toxin is removed from the body. The accent is therefore, on prevention. Tetanus toxoid provides good immunity. Passive immunization can be effected by anti-tetanus globulin (ATG). This should be given to individuals with large wounds which are contaminated by dirt, soil or foreign bodies, particularly when medical attention has not been available immediately. ATG is processed from human serum and therefore does not carry the risk of anaphylactic shock seen with tetanus anti-toxin (made in horses).

C. difficile is the cause of antibiotic-associated colitis. Antibiotic therapy may alter the gut flora and allow the growth of *C. difficile*. Certain strains produce a toxin which damages the colon, causing a spectrum of disease from mild diarrhoea to fatal colitis.

Virtually all antibiotics have caused antibiotic-associated colitis, but clindamycin, lincomycin and the newer cephalosporins are those most commonly associated with this syndrome. There is some evidence that cross infection may occur. Treatment involves stopping suspected antibiotics, and oral treatment with vancomycin or metronidazole. In severe cases colectomy may be necessary.

Gram-negative bacteria

Pseudomonas spp., *Escherichia coli* and related species

This group, which includes *Klebsiella, Enterobacter, Proteus, Serratia* and *Acinetobacter*, is responsible for the majority of infections in surgical patients. Many species are found in the gut as normal flora and cause endogenous infections following intra-abdominal surgery. They are also important causes of urinary tract infections.

These organisms are, or have the capacity to become, resistant to a wide range of antibiotics. Where broad spectrum agents such as ampicillin or cephalosporins are used widely, they will encourage the replacement of normal flora in the mouth, upper respiratory and gastro-intestinal tracts and skin with antibiotic-resistant Gram-negative species. Once established, epidemic strains of *Klebsiella* and *Acinetobacter* can effectively replace skin flora for several days. This is often found in urological, orthopaedic, neurological and cardiothoracic units, and in adult and neonatal intensive care units. Warmth, moisture and high humidity encourage environmental contamination with these Gram-negative species.

The patient who is heavily colonized with these species is prone to endogenous infection of wound site, lungs, urine and blood. He or she also acts as a focus for cross infection via the hands of staff. Urinary tract infections associated with indwelling catheters are often the earliest sign of a major cross infection with Gram-negative bacilli. Once the infection is established, the use of increasingly potent antibiotics merely reinforces the selection pressure that started the problem.

Source isolation and strict attention to hand washing and catheter care are the only means of controlling the spread of this type of infection.

Non-sporing anaerobes

As a result of improvements in isolation techniques, the importance of non-sporing anaerobes in oral, vaginal and gastro-intestinal surgery (particularly of the appendix, caecum, colon and rectum) has been fully appreciated.

Bacteroides fragilis is the main pathogen, although other *Bacteroides* spp. and fusobacteria may be involved. Very often a number of anaerobes may be isolated from an infected site. Mixed infections with anaerobes and aerobes are also common. Cross infection is not a problem. A good quality specimen, which reaches the laboratory quickly, is essential for diagnosis.

Fungal infections

Fungal infections rarely occur in surgical patients except in those who are already severely immunodepressed. They are related to the underlying disease or chemotherapy or radiotherapy rather than to surgery. The most important systemic fungal pathogens are *Candida* spp, *Aspergillus* and *Cryptococcus neoformans*. *Aspergillus* causes infection of the lungs, *C. neoformans* causes meningitis, and *Candida* spp. cause pulmonary infections and septicaemia.

Viral infections

These also are not a major problem for the normal surgical patient. Some agents, for example HBV, non-A non-B virus and cytomegalovirus (CMV) are sometimes associated with blood transfusions. Viruses of the herpes group (e.g. herpes simplex, varicella-zoster) that produce latent infections can be reactivated by any stress and may appear after operations. In the normal patient they are an inconvenience rather than a danger.

Viral infections really are only life threatening in surgical patients who are already severely immunocompromised. These patients are prone to disseminated CMV or Herpes simplex infections. The defence against these intracellular pathogens is through cell-mediated immunity, and primary or secondary defects of this system are more likely to result in serious viral infection than defects in humoral immunity.

Other infections

As with fungal and viral disease, surgical patients may get a variety of infections linked to their primary disease rather than to surgery. Many of these will be seen in transplantation surgery, including *Pneumocystis carinii* pneumonia (a protozoan), disseminated toxoplasmosis, and *Strongyloides stercoralis* infection (especially in individuals born in tropical areas such as the Carribean).

Mixed infections – microbial synergy

Infection may be caused by two or more microorganisms working synergistically. The most common example of this is the mixed infection with non-sporing anaerobes (e.g. *Bacteroides fragilis*) and facultative bacteria (e.g. *E. coli* or *Strep. faecalis*). There is good experimental evidence that such bacterial combinations can cause infection at levels well below the normal infecting dose of the individual organism. In some cases a mixed infection may resolve after treatment with a drug such as metronidazole, which is only active against anaerobic bacteria.

The basis for this type of synergy is unclear. It may be nutritional; one organism may provide essential growth factors for the other. *In vitro* some non-sporing anaerobes are able to inhibit phagocytosis and killing of bacteria such as *E. coli* or *Proteus* spp.

Bacterial–viral synergy also exists where a relatively mild virus infection can make the host susceptible to a bacterial pathogen (e.g. influenza virus and *Staph. aureus* pneumonia). This synergy may work both locally and systemically.

Microbiologists still think mainly in terms of single pathogens. The investigation of mixed infections is technically complex and still in its infancy.

This investigation leads, however, directly to the even more complex task of analysing the interactions of the normal flora with pathogens that underly such concepts as 'colonization resistance' of the gut.

Further reading

Advisory Committee on Dangerous Pathogens. *LAV/HTLV III – the causative agent of AIDS and related conditions – Revised Guidelines*. June 1986. HMSO.

Borriello P. (ed) *Antibiotic-associated Diarrhoea and Colitis*. 1984; chapters 1 and 2, Martinus Nijhoff, The Hague.

Lowbury EJL, Geddes AM, Ayliffe GAJ, Williams JD. *Control of Hospital Infection*, 1981; second edition, Chapman and Hall, London.

Report of a Combined Working Party of the Hospital Infection Society and the British Society for Antimicrobial Chemotherapy. Guidelines for the control of epidemic methicillin-resistant *Staphylococcus aureus*. *J Hosp Infect* 1986; 7:193–201.

2

Principles of microbiological diagnosis

The specimen

No amount of sophisticated microbiology will produce useful information from a poor specimen; to put it more crudely 'rubbish in, rubbish out'. A good specimen should:

(a) be truly representative of the site of infection and be sent in the correct container;
(b) arrive in the laboratory promptly or, if delayed, be stored under proper conditions;
(c) be accompanied by sufficient relevant clinical and patient information to enable the laboratory to process, interpret and return results to the correct ward or doctor.

Specimen quality

The main types of specimen from surgical patients are swabs, pus, exudate, tissue, sputum, blood and urine.

Pus, swabs, exudate and tissue

Swabs are probably the most common specimens taken from sites of infection or colonization; from superficial sites there is no real alternative. It may be necessary to moisten the swab with a little sterile water before use. When possible the swab should be sent to the laboratory in transport medium (Stuart's or Amies). This is designed to improve bacterial survival without encouraging too much growth. The use of transport medium does not, however, reduce the need for rapid transport of swabs to the laboratory.

In many situations swabs are not ideal. All too often where relatively large amounts of pus or exudate are available (e.g. at operation), a swab is merely dipped into it; this is bad practice. A good sample of fluid or purulent material will enable the laboratory to detect smaller numbers of organisms and to carry out more modern rapid diagnostic techniques that are possible to perform on a swab (e.g. gas-liquid chromatography).

Another situation in which swabs are commonly misused is when there is a discharging sinus or a lesion from which removal of superfical tissue is required and deep probing is necessary. Superficial swabs will often fail to produce the relevant pathogen and may even produce misleading results.

When exudate, pus, or tissue is sent, a reasonable quantity should be put into a suitable container. Different laboratories will vary in the type of container which they specify for such samples. Some may provide special gassed out containers for samples of pus suspected of containing anaerobic bacteria. If in doubt, always ask the laboratory.

If a sample is particularly valuable, it may be necessary to take it directly to the laboratory. Alternatively, especially in the operating theatre, the microbiologist may be able to come and take or collect the sample directly.

When samples obtained at operation need to be sent for both histopathology and microbiology remember that formalin is a highly effective antimicrobial agent as well as a fixative. Too many samples destined for microbiology inadvertently end up in formalin.

Sputum

Good sputum samples are difficult to get. If the patient is on a ventilator, a trap specimen of bronchial secretions is a good solution. Transtracheal aspiration will also provide good samples, but is not a routine procedure in Britain.

A sputum sample obtained with the help of the physiotherapist is likely to be of reasonable quality. However, the majority of sputum samples taken by non-invasive means are poor. Many samples are merely saliva. If the patient is already on antibiotics, such samples will usually grow resistant Gram-negative bacilli that are rarely significant. Some laboratories refuse to process sputum samples from patients on antibiotics on the basis that results obtained are virtually useless.

Blood

There is wide variation in the types and size of blood culture bottles. Some laboratories now use the BACTEC system in which the presence of carbon 14 in the medium allows rapid growth detection by measurement of labelled carbon dioxide. Newly appointed junior staff should check detailed instructions for the use of blood culture bottles.

The patient's skin should be disinfected with alcohol. If a needle and syringe are used, the needle should be changed before blood is put into the bottle. Contamination with skin organisms resulting from poor technique is the biggest problem encountered with blood cultures.

The problem of skin contamination has been made worse by the realization that the commonest contaminant, *Stap. epidermidis*, is now an increasingly common genuine cause of sepsis, particularly where intravenous lines are involved.

Urine

Urine is the most common specimen sent to the laboratory. Mid stream urine (MSU) samples and catheter urine (CSU) samples are the norm. Few suprapubic aspirate (SPA) samples are taken in Britain.

Too many urine samples are sent as a matter of routine without clinical indication. If the workload is increased indiscriminately in this way, there is a danger that each individual sample will receive less thorough treatment. The fact that a sample is easy to obtain does not mean that it should be sent without a good reason.

Urine is a good bacterial growth medium. With MSU samples the definition of an infection depends on the number of bacteria/ml ($> 10^5$). Contaminating organisms derived from the periurethral area can easily multiply to this level within a few hours. Therefore urine samples that cannot be sent immediately should be kept at 4° C.

The technique used to take MSU samples can also cause problems. The periurethral area can be cleaned, but only dry swabs or distilled water should be used. Antiseptics and detergents should never be used. Many antibiotics are excreted in the urine and residual antibacterial activity can persist for 2 or 3 days after ending therapy.

Transport to the laboratory

Most specimens are transported by the portering service. Even at its best this is not designed to be particularly rapid. It is quite common for several hours to pass before a sample arrives in the laboratory. This delay will be even worse if the laboratory is on a different site from the ward or department concerned.

This is an area where common sense should dictate how to handle the problem. If the specimen is urgent or important, make special arrangements for its transport. Do not assume transport medium will save the sample. Give nurses clear instructions. The responsibility for sending the sample to the laboratory rests with the clinician.

Relevant clinical/patients details

Medical staff dislike filling in request forms. These forms cannot be wholly standardized. Different pathology disciplines require different information. However, the information requested is important. Unless the patient and his/her ward or department and consultant are identified, results may go astray. Unless the requesting doctor is identified, the laboratory will not know whom to contact for further information vital for processing or interpretation.

The processing of a microbiology specimen depends on a knowledge of the relevant clinical details, the site from which the sample came and a history of recent or current antimicrobial therapy. Failure to provide this information can delay results by 24 or even 48 hours. Delegation of form filling to nurses is tempting, but often results in inadequate clinical data being given.

Specimens from patients who present a risk of infection (e.g. hepatitis B, tuberculosis) should be clearly labelled using the relevant hazard marker, so that laboratory staff can take necessary precautions. Again this is primarily the doctor's responsibility not the nurse's.

Laboratory diagnosis

The role of the laboratory is to identify organisms responsible for individual infections or outbreaks of infection and to provide details of antibiotic sensitivity patterns.

A better understanding of how a microbiology laboratory processes samples would explain much of the need for good patient information. Figure 2.1 shows briefly how a typical sample passes through the laboratory.

The laboratory is divided into sections, each of which deals with a specific type or range of specimens. How the sample is cultured, what media are used and which antibiotic sensitivities are set up, will depend on the site from which the sample came, available details about the patient and his/her other antimicrobial therapy, and any results of preliminary microscopy and other rapid diagnostic tests.

Standard microscopy, using the Gram stain, is relatively insensitive. It will show whether there is an inflammatory response (white cells in pus, sputum or urine), but may not demonstrate the causative organism. With improved immunological reagents, particularly monoclonal antibodies, immunofluorescent microscopy may be used directly on clinical material, thus improving sensitivity. Other immunological methods such as latex agglutination and enzyme immunoassays can also be used to detect microbial

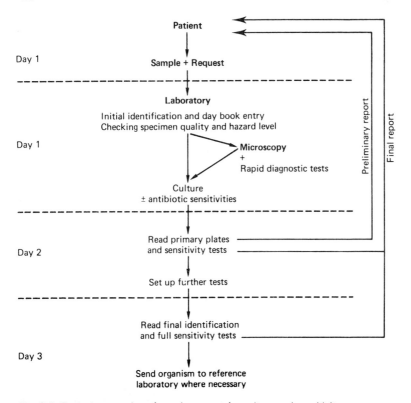

Fig. 2.1 Typical processing of specimen sent for culture and sensitivity

antigens. At present, however, relatively few bacterial species can be identified in this way (*Strep. pneumoniae, Haemophilus influenzae, Neisseria meningitides*, Group A and B beta haemolytic streptococci). No reagents are available for staphylococci, *E. coli, Pseudomonas* spp. or other Gram-negative bacilli.

In certain instances non-specific rapid diagnostic tests may be used, for example gas-liquid chromatograpy for the detection of volatile fatty acids characteristic of anaerobes and limulus lysate assay for the detection of lipopolysaccharide (endotoxin) from Gram-negative organisms. These are expensive and require special equipment or skills. They are, therefore, not widely available.

Although most organisms will grow satisfactorily within 18–24 hours, some need 48 hours incubation or longer. Anaerobes are generally slow growing, and final results may not be available for several days.

The most useful information the laboratory can provide for patient management is the antibiotic sensitivity pattern of the pathogen. In some cases identification of the organism gives the sensitivity. All group A streptococci and nearly all pneumococci will be sensitive to benzylpenicillin. In other cases it is easier and quicker to provide antibiotic sensitivities than to provide a full bacterial identification. Terms such as 'coliform' are therefore used to describe Gram-negative bacilli which could be anything from *E. coli* or *Proteus* spp. to salmonellae.

Some laboratories will provide full identification of such species only if the organism is especially resistant, when the patient is a unit where infection is a problem (e.g. virology, intensive care, burns) or if the patient is likely to stay in hospital for some time and face a series of infections. Such detailed identification is of more value in infection control surveillance than for the individual patient. Specialized serological characterization or phage typing may be referred to reference laboratories.

Few if any laboratories carry out all possible diagnostic tests. Some samples will be sent to other centres and the results of these tests will not be available so quickly unless special arrangements are made. Other tests are only economical if carried out in batches, possibly only once a week; it is as well to know when this is done. In an emergency a one off test can usually be done even if it is inordinately expensive. However, for routine patient investigation if a test is done once a week on Thursday mornings, and the specimen arrrives on Thursday afternoon, then the result will only be available 1 week later.

Apart from these problems, an interim written report should be available on the day following receipt of most samples. A full report with sensitivities should be available on 80–90 per cent of samples within 48 hours of receipt.

An increasing number of laboratories provide booklets for medical staff which explain the details of the service they provide. The key rule is to get to know the laboratory and to ask if in doubt about any sample. The surgeon who establishes a good working relationship with a laboratory, where both sides appreciate each other's problems, will get the best service. Someone who only makes contact to complain will get a correspondingly poor response.

Further reading

Stokes EJ, Ridgway GL. *Clinical Bacteriology*, 1980; fifth edition, Edward Arnold, London.

3

The nature of bacterial virulence

If bacteria have any purpose, it is to acquire nutrients so they can grow and replicate. Organisms that live on or in a host also need to avoid or resist the attempts of that host to remove or destroy them. For species with pathogenic potential these mechanisms are the primary determinants of virulence (Table 3.1).

Table 3.1 Bacterial virulence – survival and replication

Adherence to host tissue
Invasion
Acquisition of nutrients
Resistance to serum lysis
Resistance to phagocytosis
Resistance to intracellular killing
Antigenic variation

Bacterial establishment in the host

Adherence and invasion

Initially, a pathogenic organism must adhere firmly to a host surface. Adherence can result from non-specific physicochemical interactions. Bacteria with hydrophobic surfaces will adhere to cells more readily than those with hydrophilic surfaces. Specific reactions between bacterial surface ligands and cell receptors can also be involved; examples are listed in Table 3.2. Finally, extracellular material often known as 'slime' can bind bacteria, such as staphylococci, to foreign bodies and bone.

Table 3.2 Bacterial structures involved in adherence

Bacterial Species	Structure	Target cell
Group A streptococcus	Lipoteichoic acid	Buccal/pharyngeal epithelium
E. coli	K88 antigen CF/I or II	Small bowel (pig) Small bowel (man)
E. coli	P. fimbriae	Urinary epithelium
N. gonorrhoeae	Pili	Genital tract columnar epithelium
Staph. aureus	Cell wall teichoic acid	Nasal epithelium

Relatively little is known about the mechanisms of invasion. Virulent strains of invasive organisms, for example *Shigella, Yersinia* and enteroinvasive *E. coli*, are known to elaborate certain cell wall proteins not found in avirulent strains. How these function is as yet unknown.

Nutrient acquisition

If bacteria cannot acquire the necessary nutrients, they cannot grow. If the host can limit a pathogen's access to vital nutrients, this will be almost as effective a defence as direct killing of the organism.

Although many nutrients are important for bacterial growth, iron has been studied most intensively. Non-haem iron in the blood is kept at a very low level ($\leq 10^{-18}$M) because of the presence of iron-binding proteins such as transferrin and lactoferrin. These proteins have a high affinity for iron. Pathogenic bacteria have various methods of releasing and absorbing iron bound to these proteins. Similar mechanisms almost certainly exist for other essential nutrients. In animal experiments saturation of the iron-binding proteins with excess iron enhances the virulence of a wide range of bacteria.

This type of observation is important in understanding microbial pathogenicity. *In vivo* bacteria often grow in relatively harsh conditions with nutrient restriction, low oxygen tension and lowered pH. *In vitro* they are usually grown in near optimal conditions. Most bacteria can show wide variation in many of their structures in response to different growth conditions (**phenotypic variation**). Insufficient account has been taken of this variation *in vivo*, and it is likely that in many cases bacteria grown *in vitro* for the study of pathogenic mechanisms differ in vital aspects from those bacteria causing infection *in vivo*.

Resistance to serum lysis and phagocytosis

Once pathogens have breached the superficial defences, killing by phagocytic cells or by serum lysis is the host's main defence. Both complement and antibody are usually involved, although contact between bacterium and phagocyte can lead to phagocytosis.

Gram-positive bacteria are resistant to antibody/complement-mediated lysis. Gram-negative bacteria are in theory susceptible to lysis, but in practice variations in the cell envelope (presence of K antigens or changes in lipopolysaccharide or outer membrane structure) render many of them serum-resistant. Both gonococci and meningococci use the blocking antibodies present in normal human serum to prevent the action of lytic antibody and complement.

The first step in phagocytosis is the adherence of the bacterium to the phagocyte. Surface hydrophobicity will render bacteria more susceptible to phagocytosis. This can be ascertained by observing the behaviour of 'rough' and 'smooth' variants of Gram-negative organisms. They differ in the completeness of their cell lipopolysaccharide (LPS). The rough strains lack much of the outer polysaccharide part of LPS, are relatively hydrophobic and susceptible to phagocytosis. The more virulent smooth variants have more of this outer carbohydrate, which makes them less hydrophobic and less readily phagocytosed.

Even in the absence of antibody most bacterial species activate complement by the non-specific 'alternative pathway'. The possession of surface components such as sialic acid prevents this and is a useful virulence factor in the non-immune host. Examples of bacterial surface structures which inhibit phagocytosis are given in Table 3.3.

Table 3.3 Structures involved in resistance to phagocytosis

Organism	Structure
Group A streptococcus	M protein
Group B streptococcus	Sialic acid
Strep. pneumoniae	Capsular polysaccharide
H. influenzae type b	Capsular polysaccharide
Klebsiella aerogenes	Capsular polysaccharide
E. coli	Acid polysaccharide K-antigen

Resistance to intracellular killing

Some bacterial pathogens are able to survive within phagocytic cells. Any organism that can achieve this is protected from both host defences and many antimicrobial agents. In addition, the ingested organism can be carried to distant sites of the body.

The mycobacteria are the best known intracellular bacterial pathogens; *M. leprae* is the most highly adapted and to date it cannot be cultured *in vitro*. Other bacterial genera such as *Salmonella, Brucella, Listeria*, and *Chlamydia* are also intracellular pathogens. Many resulting intracellular infections are subacute or chronic, are difficult to diagnose microbiologically, require prolonged antimicrobial therapy and are prone to relapse. Highly effective antimicrobial agents such as penicillins and aminoglycosides penetrate cells poorly.

Little is known about the mechanisms of resistance to intracellular killing. Mycobacteria have thick waxy walls and might be expected to resist a hostile environment. However, genera such as *Salmonella* and *Brucella* are closely related to other bacteria that do not survive within phagocytic cells.

Antigenic variation

The immune system recognizes invading bacteria as 'non-self', and reacts accordingly to mount a response to bacterial antigen. If, however, the specificity of the bacterial antigen subsequently changes, any earlier specific immune response becomes irrelevant and the host has to start again.

Antigenic variation is most pronounced in higher organisms but it is seen in some bacteria, classically in *Borrelia recurrentis*, the cause of relapsing fever. Investigations with monoclonal probes have suggested that variations in the antigenic specificity of bacterial surface proteins may occur in other species.

Tissue damage (Table 3.4)

Once microorganisms have evaded host defences, they can damage the host by the release of potent exotoxins, by the release of toxic cell wall constituents (e.g. lipopolysaccharide) and extracellular products or, finally, by immunopathological effects. The severity of functional loss may depend on the tissue affected rather than on the degree of damage. Relatively small changes in the heart or central nervous system can have profound effects.

Table 3.4 Bacterial virulence – tissue damage

Exotoxins
Extracellular toxic products
Lipopolysaccharide
Immunopathology
antibody-mediated hypersensitivity
cell-mediated hypersensitivity

Exotoxins

Exotoxins produce their effects by acting either locally (*E. coli* and *C. difficile* enterotoxins) or at sites distant from that of infection (tetanus and diphtheria toxins). Many of these toxins consist of two units; one unit binds to cellular receptors allowing the other to penetrate the cell and produce harmful effects.

Toxic cell wall constituents

Lipopolysaccharide (LPS) endotoxin is believed to be responsible for the phenomenon of 'Gram-negative shock' which involves hypotension, thrombocytopenia, loss of peripheral vascular tone, diffuse intravascular haemolysis and deficiencies of the clotting system. Haemorrhage and inflammation occur in the lungs, kidney, liver and gastro-intestinal tract. Gram-negative shock is one of the most serious complications of Gram-negative bacterial septicaemia and causes a high mortality. Damage to the liver allows more lipopolysaccharide to enter the circulation from bacteria in the gastro-intestinal tract.

Lipopolysaccharide is a component of the outer cell wall of all Gram-negative bacteria. LPS consists of lipid A (believed to be the component responsible for toxic effects), a stable core polysaccharide region and a highly variable outer polysaccharide region. This outer part confers 'O' or 'somatic' antigen specificity to bacteria such as *E. coli*.

Lipopolysaccharide is biologically reactive as shown in Table 3.5. Its effects in Gram-negative shock are related to massive uncontrolled activation of a series of biological cascades – the complement, kinin, clotting and fibrinolytic systems. These are linked at several points and share certain common inhibitors. Lipopolysaccharide also causes endothelial damage and involves phagocytic cells and platelets.

The complexity of the reactions behind bacteriogenic shock makes effective therapy difficult. In its later phase there may be toxic damage to the myocardium.

Table 3.5 Biological activities of lipopolysaccharide

Complement activation
Activation of kinin clotting and fibrinolytic systems
Hypotension
Pyrexia
Thrombocytopenia
Transient neutropenia followed by leucocytosis
Endothelial damage
Polyclonal B cell activation

Therapy is largely supportive, maintaining adequate ventilation, tissue perfusion, acid-base and electrolyte balance, with antimicrobial therapy to counter the septicaemia. The importance of high dose corticosteroids and opiate antagonists such as naloxone is controversial. Promising results have been obtained using antiserum raised against the lipid A core polysaccharide region of LPS prophylactically and therapeutically. This is thought to neutralize the toxic effects of LPS. This work is, however, still at an early stage.

Local tissue damage by toxic extracellular products and cellular destruction

Bacteria produce a wide range of toxic extracellular products. Although these can cause serious local and systemic effects, their precise role in pathogenesis is not always clear. Examples of these products include staphylococcal haemolysins, the 'lethal toxins' of *C. perfringens* and streptococcal hyaluronidase.

Immunopathological damage

This results not from the toxic or invasive properties of the organism, but from the host's own immune response. There are four types of hypersensitivity reaction that can cause tissue damage: anaphylactic, cytotoxic, immune complex and cell-mediated hypersensitivity. The first three involve antibodies.

Anaphylactic hypersensitivity

Antigen binds to antibody (mainly IgE) already attached by its Fc region to the surface at mast cells, basophils and platelets. The cells contain vasoactive substances such as histamine, 5-hydroxytryptamine, slow-reacting substance A and chemotactic factors that are capable of stimulating acute inflammation and contracting smooth muscle. The cross linking of cell-bound IgE or IgG antibody by antigen leads to the secretion of these vasoactive agents. In mast cells this can be seen as degranulation. The precise nature of the membrane signal that controls this is not known, but it is accompanied by an influx of calcium ions and a fall in the ratio of cyclic adenosine monophosphate to cyclic guanosine monophosphate.

Local anaphylaxis in the upper or lower respiratory tract is the cause of hay fever or asthma. Systemic anaphylaxis can be fatal, massive peripheral vasodilatation leads to hypotension. Anaphylaxis is not, however, an important aspect of microbial infection, more usually being associated with reactions to pollen, serum or penicillins. Complement is not involved.

Antibody-mediated cytotoxicity

This form of immunopathology occurs when cell surface antigens are recognized by antibody. The antigens may be those of the cell or viral antigens expressed on the surface of an infected cell. Activation of complement leads to cell membrane damage and lysis. It is also possible that antibody-coated cells may be destroyed by lymphocyte-like killer (K) cells which bear Fc receptors. This phenomenon has been described *in vitro*, but its significance *in vivo* is not clear.

Cytotoxic hypersensitivity causes damage in viral infections and haemolysis in infections such as malaria and mycoplasma pneumonia, where antibodies may be formed against host red cells.

Immune complex hypersensitivity

This is the most important type of antibody-mediated immunopathology in microbial infection. Antigen antibody-antigen complexes form after an acute infection or during a subacute or chronic infection. The size and solubility of the complexes depend on the proportions of antigen and antibody present. The largest complexes are formed where there is near antigen-antibody equivalence.

Where there is antigen or, more commonly, antibody excess, small soluble complexes are formed; these circulate and end up in kidney glomeruli, skin blood vessels or joints. The immune complex activates complement and triggers an acute inflammatory response attracting neutrophils. Much of the subsequent tissue damage, haemorrhage and necrosis, results from the release of lysosomal enzymes and toxic reactive oxygen species by these cells.

Glomerulonephritis, allergic alveolitis and dengue haemorrhagic fever are manifestations of immune complex hypersensitivity following infection.

Cell-mediated hypersensitivity

In this type of hypersensitivity cellular damage is produced by T lymphocytes and macrophages rather than by antibody, complement and neutrophils. Cytotoxic T cells recognize and destroy virus infected cells. Stimulated T cells can also release a series of soluble mediators called lymphokines which modulate the activity of macrophages and monocytes. Although T cell stimulation is antigen specific, the effects of lymphokines and the subsequent activity of the macrophages are non-specific. Under the influence of lymphokines, phagocytic cells are attracted to and concentrated at sites of antigenic stimulation. Macrophages are 'activated' to a higher metabolic state. As with neutrophils, tissue damage results from the release of lysosomal enzymes.

The best example of cell-mediated hypersensitivity is seen in tuberculosis. The typical tuberculous focus has a central area of necrotic (caseous) material surrounded by mononuclear cells (lymphocytes and macrophages). Cell-mediated hypersensitivity also appears to be responsible for the skin rashes in measles and in some pox virus infections.

Immunopathological damage illustrates the fact that inappropriate or excessive immune responses may be harmful. The control mechanisms that normally limit this type of reaction are discussed more fully in Chapter 4.

4

The nature of host defences

In the normal patient there is a balance between microbial virulence and host defences. Infection occurs when this balance is upset, either when the host encounters a pathogen of high virulence or when host defence mechanisms are lowered.

Over the past 40 years the pattern of surgical infections has changed. Today most infections are caused by organisms of relatively low virulence such as staphylococci, Gram-negative enterobacteria and anaerobes, in patients with impaired defences. It is easy to think of immunocompromised patients only in terms of those with severe depression of systemic immunity. Lesser degrees of depression of host defences can, however, be significant postoperatively.

Superficial host defences – resistance versus immunity

Host resistance to infection involves not only those processes usually associated with the immune system. Many of the local superficial defences that make up the first line of defence against infection come into this category. Indeed, the involvement of systemic specific and non-specific immune mechanisms often occurs only when a pathogen has overcome first line defences.

It has already been shown that a pathogen has to adhere to host tissue if it is going to cause damage. Adherence involves the recognition of receptors in host tissue by microbial structures. If the host (or a particular host tissue) lacks these receptors, the pathogen cannot gain its initial foothold. On many epithelial surfaces the layer of mucus that overlies the cells provides a barrier to microbial adherence and invasion.

Skin

The stratified epithelium of the epidermis provides an effective mechanical barrier to pathogens. The breaching of this barrier at operation or by invasive techniques provides the basis for much surgical sepsis.

In addition to acting as a barrier, the dryness of the skin, its fatty acid content and high salt concentration all effectively limit colonization by many potential pathogens. The normal skin flora (coagulase negative staphylococci and 'diphtheroids') also acts as a defence by competing with pathogens for nutrients and by secreting antibacterial substances. 'Epidemic' strains of Gram-negative genera such as *Klebsiella* and *Acinetobacter* that have caused serious outbreaks of hospital infection are unusually resistant to normal skin defences.

Urinary tract

Urine is a good bacterial growth medium. The main defences against infection are the constant dilution and flushing of the urine and the mechanical barrier of the urethra. Women, with a short straight urethra, have more problems with urinary infection than men.

Most troublesome urinary infections can be linked to some disruption of this system, from ureteric reflux in children to anatomical or functional obstruction and incomplete bladder emptying.

Respiratory tract

The respiratory tract is lined with ciliated columnar epithelium which has many mucus-secreting goblet cells. The cilia beat upwards, moving particles trapped in the mucous layer away from the lungs. The cough reflex also removes irritant material.

Loss of ciliated epithelium, loss of cough reflex (in ventilated patients) or any obstruction to the bronchial tree, with distal pooling of secretions, can all result in pulmonary infection.

Gastro-intestinal tract

Stomach acid protects the gastro-intestinal tract against a wide range of potential pathogens. Patients with achlorhydria are more likely to develop gastro-intestinal infections. The bile salts and acids also provide a hostile environment for some high grade pathogens such as group A beta haemolytic streptococci. The role of mucus as a barrier to infection has already been mentioned.

Probably the most effective local defence is the normal flora of the gut. There is a distinction between the faecal and mucosal flora of the tract, and the faecal flora varies in different parts of the gastro-intestinal tract. Anaerobes predominate and are largely responsible for so-called 'colonization resistance' – the ability of the gut to resist the establishment of potential pathogens. Antibiotics that effect the anaerobic flora reduce this resistance and render the gut more susceptible to colonization with either primary gastro-intestinal pathogens or the antibiotic-resistant Gram-negative species that are an important cause of nosocomial infection – *Klebsiella* and *Pseudomonas*. Gastro-intestinal colonization with these genera is often the prelude to an outbreak of infection on a surgical ward. Although the concept of 'colonization resistance' seems valid, the complex bacterial interactions responsible for this effect have not been worked out.

Female genital tract

The microbial ecology of this site is as complex as that of the gut. In women of child-bearing age the normal flora consists of lactobacilli. The mucosa is rich in glycogen, and lactobacillary fermentation reduces the pH to below 4.5. This limits the growth of pathogens and effectively sets up a barrier against ascending infection. Many vaginal infections are accompanied by a change in basic vaginal flora and a rise in pH. Hormone levels may influence the capacity of pathogenic species to adhere to vaginal epithelium.

Humoral defences

Complement

The complement system consists of a series of plasma proteins that interact with one another to produce various biological effects. These are involved in both defence against infection and immunopathology. Parts of the complement system work as a biological cascade, where activation of component A produces an enzyme whose substrate is component B. When activated by A, B works on its own substrate C and so on. The clotting, fibrinolytic and kinin systems are also biological cascades; the complement system appears to be closely linked to them. All these systems can and do interact, and they share common inhibitors.

Figure 4.1 shows the essentials of the complement system without details of the individual components. Complement recognizes or can be activated either by the specific interaction between IgG or IgM antibody and antigen (**classical pathway**), or by non-specific means (**alternative pathway**). A non-specific recognition pathway is essential if complement is to function in the non-immune host. Many of the structures of the bacterial cell wall will activate the alternative complement pathway (Table 4.1). The purpose of both pathways is to produce an enzyme complex capable of activating the third component of complement, C3. C3 is the central point of the complement system, and it is the component present in highest concentration in the plasma.

C3 activation leads in turn to activation of the terminal components C5–C9 which are responsible for membrane damage and cell lysis. However, only Gram-negative bacteria are susceptible to complement-mediated lysis.

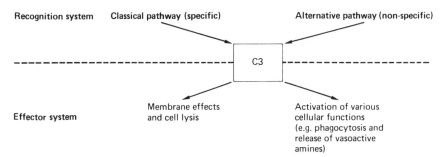

Fig. 4.1 The complement system

Table 4.1 Activators of the alternative complement pathway

Lipopolysaccharide (endotoxin)
Peptidoglycan
Polysaccharide capsules
Yeast cell walls
Aggregated immunoglobulins

Table 4.2 Biological activity of complement components

Component	Function
C3a	Release of vasoactive amines – chemotaxis
C3b	Opsonization
C5a	Release of vasoactive amines – chemotaxis
C5b	Weak opsonin
C7, 89	Membrane damage and lysis (Only Gram-negative bacteria)

More important for host defences are the biological activities of C3 and C5; these are listed in Table 4.2. C3 is split to form a large cell-bound fragment C3b and a smaller fluid phase component C3a. Activation of C5 has similar effects. C3a and C5a cause the release of vasoactive amines from mast cells and platelets. They are also strongly chemotactic for phagocytic cells, as is C3b and to a lesser degree C5b. When bound to microorganisms they act as **opsonins**. Phagocytic cells have complement receptors on their surfaces which recognize bound complement opsonin. This interaction increases the rate of microbial ingestion. Complement receptors are also involved in stimulation of oxidative killing mechanisms of the phagocyte.

Complement components are therefore involved in the stimulation of acute inflammation, allowing the defences of the intravascular compartment into the tissues. They also act as chemotactic agents attracting phagocytic cells to the site of infection. Finally, they mediate bacterial killing either by lysis or by opsonization, ingestion and intracellular destruction.

Although these processes are potent defence mechanisms, inflammation and the accumulation of phagocytic cells is also responsible for the immunopathological damage seen in immune complex diseases. Immune complexes activate complement and attract phagocytic cells. In attempting to ingest the complexes these cells release lysosomal enzymes and highly reactive oxygen radicals which damage surrounding tissue. The antigen in immune complex disease may be microbial in origin.

The complement deficiencies may be primary, as a result of a genetic deficiency of a particular component or inhibitor (thus allowing continued breakdown of a component and a consequent functional deficiency). Secondary deficiencies of the system are seen in patients with severe burns or liver disease or where there is hypercatabolism of a particular component. Deficiencies of C3, C5, C7 and C8 and the alternative pathway have all been associated with increased susceptibility to infection.

Antibodies

Antibodies are immunoglobulins. Their general structure is shown in Fig. 4.2. They consists of two long and two short polypeptide chains, the heavy and light chains. Each heavy and light chain is linked by disulphide bonds. The structure of the heavy chain determines the class of immuno-globulin; there are five classes: IgG, IgM, IgA, IgE, IgD. IgD has no direct role in antimicrobial immunity. There are four IgG subclasses IgG 1–4 and two IgA subclasses IgA 1 and 2.

Immunoglobulins are produced by B-lymphocytes in response to specific antigenic stimuli. These trigger the process of lymphocyte transformation. The lymphocyte enlarges and then undergoes several divisions to produce either a clone of identical daughter cells ready to respond to a secondary stimulus, or plasma cells which are secretory cells that produce antibodies of the same specificity as the original antigenic stimulus. B-lymphocytes are found in the spleen, lymph nodes and in the submucosal areas of the gastro-intestinal, respiratory and genital tracts.

The immunoglobulin molecule has a variable end, the Fab portion. In this portion the amino acid sequence of heavy and light chains may vary and there may be an almost infinite variety of three-dimensional shapes created by folding of the chains. The specificity of the antibody and its recognition of specific antigen is a matter of one shape fitting into another. Antibody-antigen reactions are physical not chemical reactions.

Whereas the variable Fab portion of the IgG molecule controls the anti-genic specificity of the immunoglobulin, its biological reactivity – complement activation and opsonization – is determinated by its stable Fc portion.

When a person first encounters an antigen, the resulting primary immunological response is limited by the small number of B-cells that respond to the specific stimulus. When the antigen is met again the secondary

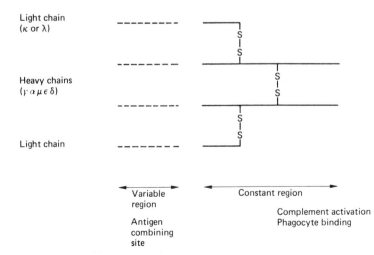

Fig. 4.2 The structure of immunoglobulin

response will be greater than the primary response, if as a result of the latter a large clone of antigen-specific B-cells exists ready to respond. Many textbooks include diagrams showing that the secondary responses are greater and appear earlier than primary ones. This latter statement is not strictly true. All antibody detection systems have a particular sensitivity. If more antibody is produced during the secondary response, this level will be exceeded earlier and the antibody response will appear to be earlier.

Not all antibodies produced are protective. Most will have no effect on the course of infection. Some may even be harmful. The ways in which antibodies protect against microbial infection are listed in Table 4.3. At mucosal surfaces IgG and secretory IgA prevent microbial adherence to epithelium and neutralize toxins. IgG and IgM antibodies can both neutralize viruses and Lyse Gram-negative bacteria. These two classes of antibody also act as opsonins to promote phagocytosis and intracellular killing. Activation of complement through the classical pathway facilitates acute inflammation whereby humoral and cellular defences can be moved from vascular to extravascular sites and concentrated at the site of infection. IgE has no protective function against bacteria and viruses but together with eosinophils provides a defence against some parasitic infections.

Table 4.3 Protective function of antibody

Virus neutralization
Prevention of adherence
Toxin neutralization
Stimulation of acute inflammation
Bacterial lysis
Opsonization

Although antibody and complement are the major opsonins, other molecules found in plasma may also function in this way. Fibronectin is a high molecular weight glycoprotein that binds to surface components of a range of organisms, including *Staph. aureus* and beta haemolytic streptococci. Fibronectin mediates the attachment of bacteria to cells and other surfaces and has some opsonic activity; the clinical importance of this is unclear. Tuftsin is a tetrapeptide derived from a non-specific immunoglobulin made in the spleen. It also promotes phagocytosis, and it is absent in splenectomized patients. Although they are prone to infection, the role of tuftsin in the normal individual is, as with fibronectin, not clear.

Nutritional factors

There is good clinical evidence that general malnutrition reduces resistance to infection. *Pneumocystis carinii* pneumonia, now closely associated with immunosuppressed patients, particularly those with Acquired Immunodeficiency Syndrome (AIDS), is also seen in malnourished children. Surgical patients, particularly those with advanced malignancy or with major gastrointestinal problems, can be included in this group. Little is known, however, about the mechanisms of reduced resistance to infection seen in malnutrition and the role of individual nutrients.

Severe nutritional deficiency affects humoral and cell-mediated immunity, phagocytosis and the integrity of mucosal surfaces.

Vitamins

Vitamin A, B and C deficiency all affect mucosal surfaces, thereby reducing this first line of defence against infection. In experimental animals vitamin A deficiency decreases resistance to *Pseudomonas, Candida* and *M. tuberculosis*. The role of vitamin C in resistance to infection remains controversial. The use of this vitamin in clinical trials has largely failed to substantiate this role, although animal work with streptococci and staphylococci has proved more promising. Vitamin C can potentiate neutrophil chemotaxis and hexose monophosphate shunt activity which are important in phagocytosis and oxidative killing respectively.

Metals

Iron, zinc and copper are associated with resistance to infection.

Bacteria need iron for growth. In the host the high affinity of iron-binding proteins (transferrin, lactoferrin) for non-haem iron means that as long as these proteins remain unsaturated they keep the level of free iron too low for bacterial growth. Only those bacteria with mechanisms for releasing this iron survive. Experimentally, iron overload potentiates a range of infections. There is, however, a paradox here because a number of studies have shown that iron deficiency can also result in increased susceptibility to infection. In these patients both lymphocyte and neutrophil function was impaired. It seems that the similar effects of iron overload and iron deficiency are expressed through different mechanisms.

Less is known about zinc and copper. A zinc peptide complex found in amniotic fluid seems to have a broad spectrum of antibacterial activity.

Cellular immunity

Phagocytosis

Phagocytic cells may be mononuclear (monocytes and macrophages) or polymorphonuclear (neutrophils and eosinophils). In addition to cells circulating in the blood, in the tissues or in bone marrow reserves, there are fixed cells of the mononuclear phagocyte system, including Kupffer cells of the liver. As these fixed cells cannot be isolated easily and studied *in vitro*, their importance tends to be overlooked. Phagocytosis by these cells, particularly in liver and spleen, plays an important role, however, in clearing the blood of bacteria and other microorganisms.

To function, phagocytic cells have to move into the tissue where most infections originate. The acute inflammatory response allows them to do this. As the post-capillary venules dilate and the blood flow slows, neutrophils and monocytes begin to adhere to the endothelial lining of the vessels. During acute inflammation the endothelial cells contract to leave gaps through which the motile phagocytic cells move out into the tissue. The ability to adhere and move randomly are key properties of phagocytic cells which can be measured.

This random movement can be directed by chemical signals giving rise to chemotaxis. Chemotactic agents may be derived from the host (including C3a and C5a) or from the pathogen. Their effect is to concentrate neutrophils and, later, macrophages at the site of maximal chemical stimulus (i.e. the site of infection).

Ingestion of particles by phagocytic cells occurs as a result of contact. If the particle is hydrophobic, its adherence to the phagocyte membrane will be enhanced. The process of ingestion is increased if host components bound to the microbial surface are recognized by receptors on the phagocyte membrane. This process is known as opsonization. As described above, the main opsonins are IgG and IgM antibodies and C3b. The energy which the cell needs for ingestion is derived from glycolysis and therefore does not need oxygen. To kill ingested bacteria, however, phagocytic cells use both oxidative and non-oxidative mechanisms (Table 4.4). The process of killing is quite separate from that of ingestion. In some congenital diseases, particularly chronic granulomatous disease, microbial ingestion by phagocytic cells is normal, but killing almost entirely absent.

Table 4.4 Phagocytic killing mechanisms

Oxidative	Non-oxidative
Peroxides	Cationic proteins
Superoxide	Acid hydrolases
Singlet oxygen	Low pH
Hydroxyl radical	Lactoferrin

Once the bacterium is killed, it must be digested. Failure to degrade microbial components may result in excessive antigenic stimulation by these components and subsequent immunopathological damage.

Cell-mediated immunity

The host defences described so far cannot deal with pathogens capable of surviving within cells; cell-mediated mechanisms are required for this. The key cell is the thymus-dependent or T-lymphocyte. T-lymphocytes are long lived, and they constantly circulate from the arterial system to the lymphatics and back to the venous system via the thoracic duct. They can be defined by the presence of cell surface markers and the different types can be subdivided in the same way.

T-cells have both regulatory and effector functions (Table 4.5). Regulation of the immune response is effected by T-helper and T-suppressor cells which can control both humoral and cell-mediated response. As described above in the section on immunopathology, the immune response can cause considerable tissue damage unless excessive or inappropriate responses are controlled.

T-cells stimulated by specific antigen enlarge and then divide to generate memory cells, cytotoxic T-cells, or T-cells which release a series of soluble factors (**lymphokines**) that modulate the activity of mononuclear phagocytes (Table 4.6).

Table 4.5 T-cell functions

Helper cells	⎫
Suppressor cells	⎬ Regulate cell-mediated and humoral responses
	⎭
Cytotoxicity	
Delayed hypersensitivity and release of lymphokines	

Table 4.6 Lymphokines

Chemotactic factors
Migration inhibition factor
Macrophage activating factor
Gamma interferon
Mitogenic factors
Cytotoxic factors
Lymphocyte inhibitory factor

Cytotoxic T-cells recognize antigen on the surface of target cells, bind to them and kill them. The target may be a microbial antigen expressed on the surface of an infected cell. This is important in viral infections. T-cells from an individual will, however, only kill virus-infected target cells carrying the same major histocompatibility antigens, suggesting that they also play a part in this process.

Many intracellular microbial pathogens can survive within normal macrophages. Stimulated T-cells release lymphokines which not only attract and concentrate macrophages at the site of infection, but also activate them, boosting their metabolic activity and enabling them to kill ingested pathogens that would otherwise have survived. Although T-cell stimulation by microorganisms is specific, the activated macrophages function nonspecifically.

Among the lymphokines is immune or gamma interferon. This can protect against infection by rendering cells non-permissive for viral replication. It may also enhance the activity of another group of mononuclear cells, the natural killer (NK) cells. NK cells can destroy cells infected with intracellular pathogens.

Cell-mediated reactivity can be assessed *in vivo* by skin tests. Intradermal injection of antigen stimulates a delayed skin reaction which is maximal at 48–72 hours with a mononuclear cell infiltrate. *In vitro* techniques include lymphocyte transformation by antigens or T-cell mitogens (phytohaemagglutinin – PHA) and the inhibition of macrophage migration by antigen-stimulated T-cells.

Interaction of host defences

As can be seen from the preceding sections, few individual defence mechanisms work in isolation. At the mucosal surface mucus, cilia, secretory IgA and phagocytic cells all play a part in protection against microbial invasion. Antibodies and complement work together to lyse bacteria and to produce effective opsonization. The efficiency of non-specific phagocytosis is focused and enhanced by humoral opsonins and by antibody- and complement-mediated acute inflammation. Cell-mediated immune defences against bacteria depend on T-cell/macrophage interactions.

Co-operation between elements of the immune system also works at the level of initiation and control. Lymphocytes respond best to antigens presented by cells of the macrophage line. Regulatory lymphocytes provide the fine tuning of the system.

Immunodeficiency

Immunodeficiency can be congenital or acquired. Congenital defects are rare; they do, however, reveal important information about the type of organisms that are controlled by particular elements of the immune system (Table 4.7).

Table 4.7 Infections associated with primary immunodeficiency

Immune defect	Types of infection
C3	Pyogenic
C7–9	Gonococci and meningococci
Myeloid cells	Pyogenic especially catalase-positive organisms (e.g. staphylococci)
T-cells	Mycobacteria, Candida, virus infections, particularly herpes
B-cells	Pyogenic, especially capsulated organisms (e.g. pneumococci)

When managing patients with acquired immunodeficiency, effective empirical chemotherapy is crucial for successful treatment of infection. If the elements of the immune system which are most likely to be affected are known, it is possible to determine the most likely type of infecting organisms against which empirical therapy should be directed.

Following surgery there is often a temporary abnormality in phagocytic cell function, particulary chemotaxis. Cell-mediated immunity may also be affected, and in surgical patients there is evidence that inhibition of delayed hypersensitivity skin responses may indicate a group of patients who are particularly susceptible to infection. It is not known whether there is a direct link, or the skin response is merely a useful marker for another defect.

Burns and other major trauma affect the levels of immunoglobulin and complement as well as phagocytic function. Thus in addition to providing a suitable site of entry for pathogens, this type of injury makes the individual prone to infection.

Diabetes mellitus has marked effects on acute inflammation and phagocytic function, secondary to hyperglycaemia. Unfortunately, both the stress of surgery and that of infection often worsens the diabetes, creating a vicious circle.

Invasive malignancies of any type can result in severe immunodeficiency, either from invasion of the marrow, from the chemotherapy or radiotherapy used to manage the condition, or secondary to the malnutrition that often accompanies malignancy. Malabsorption and malnutrition may play a part in major gastro-intestinal surgery.

Further reading

Dick G. (ed) *Immunological Aspects of Infectious Diseases*, 1979; Medical and Technical Press, Lancaster.

Mims CA. *The Pathogenesis of Infectious Disease*, 1982; second edition, Academic Press, London.

5

Antimicrobial agents

Antimicrobial agents can be used in three areas which are relevant to surgery.

- To decontaminate inanimate objects (instruments and endoscopes)
- As topical agents on skin and mucous membranes
- As oral and parenteral chemoprophylaxis or therapy

Chemical disinfection/sterilization of inanimate surfaces

Disinfection is the selective removal of pathogenic organisms, whereas sterilization is the destruction of all vegetative organisms and spores.

Disinfection should be distinguished from cleaning. Dust and dirt do not always equal significant microbial contamination, and too much disinfection of surfaces is done in hospitals where simple cleaning would be sufficient.

Chemical disinfection is not instantaneous. The degree of microbial killing will depend on the concentration of disinfectant and the exposure time. The presence of blood or other organic material inactivates some disinfectants. Surfaces should be cleaned before being disinfected. This is particularly important with complex instruments.

The main groups of disinfectants currently used for decontaminating inanimate objects and surfaces are listed in Table 5.1.

Table 5.1 Main antimicrobial agents used for disinfecting inanimate surfaces

Category	Example	Comment
Phenols	Hycolin	
Halogens	Sodium hypochlorite	Good viricidal and sporicidal activity but corrodes metal surfaces
Aldehydes	Glutaraldehyde	Good viricidal and sporicidal activity but can cause sensitization
Alcohols	Isopropyl alcohol	Optimum concentration 70%
Quaternary ammonium compounds	Cetrimide	Relatively poor activity Good cleansing agent

Phenolics are good general purpose agents but have limited activity against viruses. For these organisms hypochlorite and glutaraldehyde are the most effective agents, and they should be used where blood spillage occurs in patients carrying HBV or HIV. Glutaraldehyde is used for treating heat-sensitive instruments such as cystoscopes and bronchoscopes, and it is probably the closest that a chemical agent can come to providing true sterilization. However, a long exposure time (60 minutes) must be allowed for this, and the instrument must be clean. Sensitization caused by repeated exposure to glutaraldehyde can be a problem among nurses.

In general, chemical agents should only be used for sterilization when heat or gaseous sterilization cannot be used. Correct concentration, temperature, pH and exposure times are vital.

Disinfection of skin, wounds and mucous surfaces

Although some agents (e.g. alcohol) mentioned above can be used on living tissue, toxicity excludes many others (Table 5.2). Hand-washing, skin and mucous surface preparation before surgery and the disinfection of traumatic (or surgical) wounds are of major importance.

Table 5.2 Antimicrobial agents used in skin, wound and mucous membrane disinfection

Category	Examples	Comment
Alcohols	Ethyl alcohol	Optimum concentration 70%
	Isopropyl alcohol	Very rapid action
Bis phenols	Hexachlorophane	More active against Gram-positive than against Gram-negative organisms
Biguanides	Chlorhexidine	Cumulative effect Activity reduced in presence of serum and blood
Quaternary ammonium	Cetrimide	Useful cleansing agent
Halogens	Iodine	Some sporicidal activity
	Povidone iodine	
Silver compounds	Silver nitrate	Useful in burns

To understand the use of these agents, particularly on the skin, it is necessary to see the nature of the challenge. The skin has a natural resident flora and a transient flora. The resident flora is largely Gram-positive, consisting of coagulase-negative staphylococci and aerobic and anaerobic corynebacteria (diphtheroids). The constituents of the resident flora change, depending on the anatomical site and whether the individual works in a hospital. In the nose, axilla, groin and perineum *Staph. aureus* may be found normally in 15–30 per cent of the population and in these sites and the forehead total bacterial counts will be higher.

The transient flora includes organisms with considerable pathogenic potential, (e.g. *Staph. aureus*, beta haemolytic streptococci and *Candida* spp.) together with others of lesser virulence, particularly Gram-negative species such as *E. coli* and *Pseudomonas* spp. The picture is complicated by the fact that a few epidemic strains of Gram-negative organisms, for example *Klebsiella* and *Acinetobacter*, can colonize the skin in the long term and effectively become part of the resident flora.

Handwashing

There are three levels of hand hygiene. First, social handwashing which should be carried out to remove dirt and gross contamination; for this soap and water are sufficient. Secondly, hygienic handwashing is required prior to carrying out wound dressings and minor procedures on the wards and between examining patients. The third level is surgical handwashing. For both hygienic and surgical handwashing antiseptic preparations are necessary. The biguanide chlorhexidine and the iodophor, povidone iodine, are the most commonly used preparations; both are available as aqueous detergents for handwashing, chlorhexidine as a 4 per cent preparation, povidone iodine as a 10 per cent preparation. Alternatively 3 per cent detergent hexachlorophane can be used; this is particularly active against staphylococci. In busy units such as intensive care wards, repeated handwashing may not always be practicable, and here the use of an alcohol-based chlorhexidine preparation (0.5 per cent chlorhexidine gluconate in 70 per cent isopropyl alcohol) that can be used as a hand rub is an alternative. A bottle of such a preparation can be put by each bed. The alcohol adds to the bactericidal action of the chlorhexidine.

Disinfection of skin and operation sites

Iodine, iodophors and chlorhexidine are all used for skin preparation. Quaternary ammonium compounds such as cetrimide are often available in casualty departments and operating theatres but, even when combined with chlorhexidine, they should only be used for cleaning dirty wounds and skin prior to proper skin disinfection. The most effective skin preparations are alcohol-based – 0.5 per cent chlorhexidine, 10 per cent povidone-iodine or 1 per cent iodine, all in 70 per cent alcohol.

Spores are resistant to alcohols and chlorhexidine, but are susceptible to povidone iodine provided the exposure time is long enough (30 minutes). *C. perfringens* spores from the gastro-intestinal tract may contaminate the skin of the buttocks and upper thighs. In operations on these areas (such as hip replacements and above knee amputations), sporicidal skin preparation with an iodophor may be of use, although it cannot replace the need for prophylactic antibiotics.

Disinfection of mucous membranes

Alcoholic preparations are contra-indicated. Aqueous preparations of both chlorhexidine and povidone iodine can, however, be used in low concentrations. Special formulations are available for use in the mouth and vagina, and dilute solutions have been used in wounds. Chlorhexidine can also be used for bladder washouts.

The nose is a common site for *Staph. aureus* carriage and 1 per cent chlorhexidine cream sometimes combined with neomycin has been used to eradicate carriage. Care must be taken with the neomycin as it can stimulate resistance not only to this antibiotic, but also to gentamicin and other aminoglycosides.

A novel topical antimicrobial, mupirocin (pseudomonic acid), is now available. This is primarily designed for use on skin, but a formulation is being developed for nasal use. Mupirocin has been shown to be effective against the epidemic multi-resistant strains of *Staph. aureus* currently causing serious cross infection problems worldwide.

Burns

Large areas of burned skin present special problems. Burns are highly susceptible to infection with beta haemolytic streptococci, *Pseudomonas* spp. and other Gram-negative bacteria. Silver preparations such as silver nitrate and silver sulphadiazine creams have been used successfully for topical chemoprophylaxis.

Systemic antimicrobial agents

The first widely effective systemic antimicrobial agents were the sulphonamides introduced in 1935. The first antibiotic (an antimicrobial produced by a microorganism rather than a chemist) was benzylpenicillin, described by Fleming in 1929, but not purified until 1940 by Florey and Chain.

Antimicrobial agents can be divided into those that kill bacteria at sufficiently high concentration (**bactericidal**), and those that merely inhibit growth (**bacteriostatic**). Some bacteriostatic agents are highly effective. Most antimicrobial therapy does not aim to kill all invading organisms, but rather to restore the balance between host defences and microbial invasion in favour of the host. Host defences then complete the task. This is why severely immunocompromised patients often respond poorly to chemotherapy. When antimicrobial agents are viewed in this way, prevention of bacterial growth may be just as effective as bacterial killing.

Sensitivity to antimicrobial agents is usually tested by disc diffusion techniques, in which antibiotics impregnated on a filter paper disc diffuse out and inhibit the surrounding growth of sensitive organisms, but not that of resistant organisms. Sometimes a quantitative measure of antimicrobial activity is required and this is expressed as either the minimum inhibitory concentration (MIC) or the minimum bactericidal concentration (MBC).

The antibiotic sensitivity report provided by the bacteriology laboratory is based on *in vitro* testing. It is, however, only one factor in considering the clinical effectiveness of chemotherapy. The other factors are listed in Table 5.3. Some useful rules are given below.

Table 5.3 Assessment of antimicrobial agent

In vitro activity against organism
Pharmacokinetics – tissue and cell penetration
Spectrum of activity
Toxicity and therapeutic index
Capacity to stimulate microbial resistance
Cost

- If a patient is responding to therapy and the laboratory report suggests the organism is resistant, follow the patient not the form.
- If the antibiotic appears to be effective *in vitro* but the patient is not responding, remember to check that dosage and route of administration are adequate. Too many seriously ill patients are given inadequate oral therapy.
- Do not expect antimicrobial agents to be successful in the presence of an undrained abscess or effusion, a foreign body or poor vascular perfusion. The answer may be surgical correction of the underlying problem rather than a change of antibiotic.

Individual groups of antimicrobial agents

Penicillins

The penicillins are bactericidal antibiotics that act on the bacterial cell wall. Benzylpenicillin and the acid stable phenoxymethyl penicillin are the only wholly naturally produced members of the group. They are narrow spectrum agents active only against Gram-positive genera (staphylococci, streptococci and clostridia) and gonococci and meningococci. All other penicillins are semi-synthetic. This means that the 6 amino penicillanic acid structure is produced microbiologically and the amino group is then substituted synthetically (Fig. 5.1). This is the process that was worked out by Chain in collaboration with Beechams in the 1950s, it and opened the way for the multitude of semi-synthetic penicillins now available. Table 5.4 lists the main agents in this group and their spectrum of activity.

Penicillins are only toxic in high doses, when they can cause bleeding, or if given intrathecally in normal systemic doses, when they can cause convulsions and death. The main danger is hypersensitivity ranging from skin rashes to full anaphylaxis. The rash that sometimes follows ampicillin therapy (particularly in cases of glandular fever) is not true penicillin hypersensitivity.

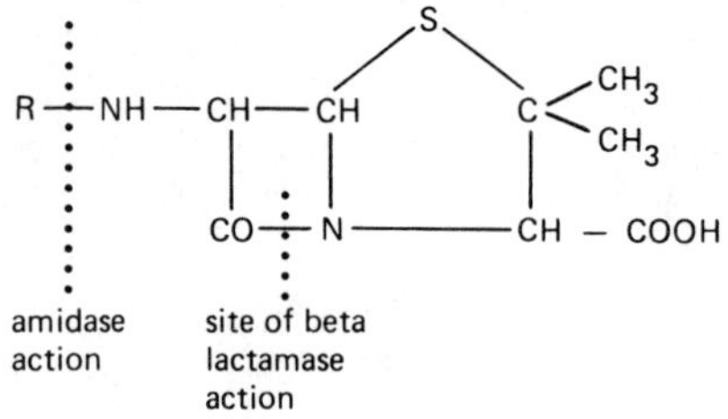

amidase action

site of beta lactamase action

R   Synthetic group can be substituted here after amidase treatment of 6 APA nucleus produced in culture by *Penicillium chrysogenum*. Structure of R will determine spectrum of activity and pharmacokinetic properties of the penicillin.

Fig. 5.1 6-amino penicillanic acid (6-APA) nucleus: the basis of semi-synthetic penicillins

Table 5.4 Semisynthetic penicillins

Antibiotic	Spectrum of activity	Comment
Ampicillin and amoxycillin	Broad – not pseudomonas	Not penicillinase stable
Methicillin Cloxacillin Flucloxacillin	Penicillinase-producing staphylococci	Methicillin not an oral agent Flucloxacillin better absorbed orally than cloxacillin
Carbenicillin Ticarcillin	Broad – including pseudomonas	Disodium salts High dosage needed: 15–40 g/day
Mezlocillin Azlocillin Piperacillin	Broad – including pseudomonas	Monosodium salts Dosage 12–15 g/day

Cephalosporins

These are closely related to penicillins: they share the beta lactam ring and have a similar mode of action. Unlike the penicillins the cephalosporin nucleus can be substituted at two sites giving even greater scope for variation; in recent years this has been fully exploited.

With the exception of cephalexin and cephradine, most cephalosporins cannot be given orally. They are often divided into first, second and third generation compounds (Table 5.5). The second and third generation agents are progressively more resistant to destruction by penicillinases and cephalosporinases produced by Gram-negative organisms. In addition many third generation cephalosporins have significant anti-pseudomonal activity.

Table 5.5 Cephalosporins

First generation	Second generation	Third generation
Cephalothin Cephaloridine Cephalexin Cephradine Cefazolin Cefaclor	Cefuroxime Cefamandole Cefoxitin*	Cefotaxime Cefsulodin Ceftazidime Ceftizoxime Cefotetan Ceftriaxone Latamoxef*

*Cefoxitin and latamoxef are not true cephalosporins but they are closely related

This increasing activity against Gram-negative species is, however, associated with a reduced activity against staphylococci, and third generation cephalosporins should not be used in staphylococcal infections. **All cephalosporins are inactive against enterococci.**

Cephalosporins can be nephrotoxic, particularly if combined with diuretics such as frusemide and ethacrynic acid or with aminoglycoside antibiotics. Although the newer agents are largely excreted in the urine, some of them have significant biliary excretion. In this way they reach the colon, and some of the problems associated with the newer cephalosporins (bleeding and antibiotic-associated colitis) may result from their effects on the normal flora of the colon. It is estimated that 10 per cent of patients allergic to penicillins will also be allergic to cephalosporins.

Aminoglycosides

These are bactericidal antibiotics that act on protein synthesis at the ribosome. They are not absorbed from the gastro-intestinal tract, and therefore have to be given intravenously or intramuscularly. Streptomycin was the first aminoglycoside to be discovered, in 1942. It is now used largely for treating tuberculosis. The important aminoglycosides are gentamicin, tobramycin, netilmicin and amikacin, all of which are ototoxic and nephrotoxic. Excretion is almost entirely renal and patients with renal impairment can easily experience problems. Therapy should be monitored by measuring serum levels and assessing renal function. It is claimed that netilmicin is less toxic than the others.

Aminoglycosides are active against staphylococci and most Gram-negative bacilli including *Pseudomonas*. They are inactive against anaerobes and have poor activity against streptococci and *Haemophilus* spp.

Generally, gentamicin and tobramycin are used as first line aminoglycosides; netilmicin is an alternative, particularly if toxicity is a major worry. Amikacin should be reserved for organisms that are resistant to other aminoglycosides.

The dosage of gentamicin given should be based on age, sex, weight and renal function. The idea of a fixed dose of 80 mg t.d.s. is still prevalent. In many cases this dose will result in inadequate therapy which is usually a greater problem than overdosing and toxicity.

Aminoglycosides have relatively poor tissue penetration: a serum level of 8–10 mg/litre may produce a level of only 2–3 mg/litre in the sputum of a patient with pneumonia. The aim should be to reach peak serum concentrations of 10–12 mg/litre (higher concentrations may cause problems of toxicity) and a trough of < 2 mg/litre.

Chloramphenicol, tetracyclines and erythromycin

These agents are bacteriostatic and act on protein synthesis at the ribosome. Unlike the beta lactam antibiotics and the aminoglycosides, they are lipid-soluble and have excellent tissue and cell penetration.

Chloramphenicol can cause irreversible marrow depression. It should therefore only be used for certain conditions such as typhoid, *Haemophilus influenzae* infections and neonatal meningitis. It is not a drug that should normally be needed for treating surgical patients; this is also true for tetracyclines and erythromycin. They are useful in the treatment of mycoplasma and chlamydial infections, erythromycin is specific for legionella pneumonia, and they can substitute for penicillin in sensitive patients. They are rarely needed for the seriously ill surgical patient.

Vancomycin

This antibiotic is bactericidal and acts on cell wall synthesis. It is not absorbed from the gut and has a narrow spectrum of activity limited to Gram-positive bacteria. Vancomycin must be given intravenously and can cause tissue damage if it leaks out of the vessels. It is also nephrotoxic and ototoxic, and patients' serum levels need to be monitored. Excretion is largely renal and, as with aminoglycosides, patients with impaired renal function are likely to suffer problems.

With the increasing importance of *Staph. epidermidis* and the appearance of epidemic methicillin-resistant *Staph. aureus* sensitive only to vancomycin, the drug is now used more commonly. Vascular, cardiothoracic and orthopaedic surgeons in particular may need to use vancomycin more often in the future. Fortunately, staphylococci and streptococci show no signs of becoming resistant to vancomycin. A related compound, teichoplanin, is undergoing clinical trials. It has a similar spectrum of activity, but improved pharmacokinetics.

Oral vancomycin is the drug of choice for treating antibiotic-associated colitis caused by *Clostridium difficile.*

Lincomycin and clindamycin

Both these agents are bactericidal drugs that act on protein synthesis. They are active against Gram-positive bacteria and have good cell and tissue penetration. They are also highly active against anaerobes.

Lincomycin and clindamycin are the two drugs most commonly linked with antibiotic-associated colitis. They have certainly caused a number of fatal cases, some of which were associated with usage for trivial complaints such as upper respiratory tract infections. They are, however, good antibiotics for anaerobic infections and for staphylococcal infections in bone. For serious sepsis of this type, risks should be balanced against benefits.

Rifampicin and fusidic acid

Rifampicin is a broad spectrum antibiotic which is well absorbed and distributed. It has been used mainly for treating tuberculosis but is also effective against resistant staphylococci. It should never be used on its own as resistance develops rapidly. Excretion is largely hepatic and it can cause liver damage. Its role is that of a second or third line agent for dealing with clearly defined sepsis.

Fusidic acid is a narrow-spectrum agent whose only clinical role is in the treatment of staphylococcal sepsis. As with rifampicin, it should not be used on its own because of the rapid emergence of resistance. It is normally given with an anti-staphylococcal penicillin such as flucloxacillin.

Polymixins

Polymixin and colistin are peptides that attack the bacterial cell membrane. They are not absorbed from the gut, and are therefore used for selective bowel decontamination. They are only active against Gram-negative species. Before the advent of aminoglycosides they were the only agents active against *Pseudomonas*, but now they are rarely used systemically.

Non-antibiotic antibacterial agents

The most important synthetic antibacterial agents are the sulphonamides and trimethoprim, nitroimidazoles, quinolones and nitrofurans.

Sulphonamides and trimethoprim

Sulphonamides and trimethoprim interfere with the conversion of para-aminobenzoic acid to folic acid and folic acid to folinic acid respectively. Folate synthesis is necessary for the production of nucleotides and hence nucleic acid. Sulphonamides and trimethoprim both have a broad spectrum of activity and, although bacteriostatic, exhibit synergy when combined. This combination (co-trimoxazole) is in the ratio of five parts of sulphamethoxazole to one part of trimethoprim. The pharmacokinetics, cell and tissue penetration of both the combination and its two components are good. Trimethoprim has few side-effects, apart from causing folate deficiency and megaloblastic anaemia, but sulphonamides can cause renal damage, hypersensitivity reactions (Stevens Johnson syndrome), agranulocytosis, haemolytic anaemia and hepatitis. Trimethoprim is effective on its own, particularly for urinary tract infections.

Nitroimidazoles

The nitroimidazoles, metronidazole and tinidazole are, with a few exceptions, active only against anaerobic bacteria. They are well absorbed by the oral and rectal routes; intravenous administration should be reserved for circumstances in which the other routes are inappropriate. Tissue distribution is good. To date, despite extensive (and in some cases inappropriate) use for pre-operative prophylaxis, little evidence of bacterial resistance has been seen. Nitroimidazoles have have few serious side-effects but often make patients feel unwell. Patients should not take alcohol as the combination can produce a disulfuram-like effect.

Quinolones

The quinolones are a group of antibacterial agents, modifications of which are currently undergoing evaluation. They act on DNA gyrases, enzymes responsible for the supercoiling of bacterial chromosomal DNA. Until recently only nalidixic acid was in general use. It is only effective as a urinary antiseptic with no activity against *Pseudomonas*, staphylococci or streptococci. New quinolone compounds are now undergoing clinical trials. These include ciprofloxacin and norfloxacin, which have shown promise as therapy for systemic infections and are active against Gram-negative bacilli with some activity against staphylococci. None is yet released for general use in the UK.

Nitrofurans

As with nalidixic acid, nitrofurans such as nitrofurantoin are urinary anti-septics that act on bacterial DNA. They only act well at acid pH, and are therefore of little value when the urine is alkaline. They are broad spectrum agents and have been used at low dosage for the long-term prevention of recurrent urinary tract infections. Peripheral neuropathy can be caused in patients with poor renal function.

Antifungal agents

Systemic fungal infection is rare except in the severely immunocompromised patient. Superficial mycoses, however, are common, *Candida* being the main genus. Such infection often results from therapy with broad spectrum antibiotics.

Nystatin is a polyene antibiotic which acts upon the cell membrane. It is active against *Candida*, but has been superseded as a systemic agent by newer compounds. It is used for suppressing gastro-intestinal, oral and vaginal candidiasis.

The other main polyene antifungal is amphotericin B. This is still standard therapy for systemic candidiasis, cryptococcal and aspergillus infections. Unfortunately, amphotericin B, which is given intravenously, is often toxic, causing fever, nausea, thrombophlebitis, hypokalaemia and renal damage. It is, however, still the most reliable therapy for serious fungal diseases.

Other antifungal agents include 5-fluorocytosine.This is useful for *Candida* and cryptococcal infections but cannot be relied upon as monotherapy and it is usually combined with amphotericin B.

The imidazoles, miconazole and ketoconazole, are other useful antifungal agents. Ketoconazole, when combined with fluorocytosine or amphotericin B, has a low toxicity and an additive effect against *Candida* and *Cryptococcus*.

Antiviral agents

As viruses live within host cells and use the mechanisms of the host cell to replicate, the problem has always been how to kill the virus without damaging the cell.

The main antiviral compounds are listed in Table 5.6. Agents such as iododeoxyuridine, cytosine arabinoside and adenine arabinoside act by inhibiting nucleic acid synthesis.

Table 5.6 Antiviral agents

Drug	Infection
Acyclovir	Herpes simplex and varicella-zoster (cytomegalovirus)
Amantidine	Influenza and herpes simplex
Iododeoxyuridine	Herpes simplex and varicella-zoster (cytomegalovirus)
Adenine arabinoside	Herpes simplex and varicella-zoster (cytomegalovirus)
Interferons	Broad range of viruses

The most promising new compound, acyclovir, is unfortunately active only against some herpes viruses. It enters the cell and is converted to the active triphosphate. This inhibits viral DNA polymerase while leaving the equivalent host enzyme largely unaffected. Acyclovir is effective against herpes simplex and varicella-zoster. Derivatives are now being developed which may be active against other herpes viruses.

Amantadines act by blocking viral entry into host cells. They have been used for prophylaxis and therapy of influenza.

Interferons are produced by infected cells and by T-lymphocytes. They reduce the susceptibility of other target cells to infection. To date the high cost of producing interferons has limited their use. Even with modern culture and molecular biological techniques they are still expensive and, although they appear to be effective antiviral agents, their final clinical role remains unclear.

Major advances in antiviral chemotherapy are likely to occur within the next 5 years. Their impact will, however, be mainly in transplant surgery where viral infections are one of the main limits to success.

Monitoring of antimicrobial therapy

Antimicrobial therapy needs to be monitored for toxicity and efficacy, both when agents with a low therapeutic index are being used (aminoglycosides, chloramphenicol and vancomycin) and when therapy is being pushed to its limits, (e.g. in treatment of bacterial endocarditis).

Serum level

Measurement of serum levels is mandatory when aminoglycosides and vancomycin are being used, and preferable when chloramphenicol is being given to young infants. Levels can be measured by bioassay or by chemical or immunological assay. The latter two are more costly but more rapid so that results are available well before the next dose of antibiotic is due.

The principle is simple. Blood is taken immediately before a dose is due and 30–60 minutes after the dose has been taken. The level in the first sample gives the trough concentration and the level in the second gives the peak concentration. For the system to work, dose intervals should be spaced evenly. Table 5.7 shows necessary trough and peak levels of the main antimicrobial agents needed to avoid toxicity. In those agents that are excreted by the kidney, renal function should be monitored by measuring creatinine clearance or serum creatinine; serum urea measurement is inadequate.

VIIIth cranial nerve function

For long-term (more than 1 week) treatment by aminoglycosides and vancomycin an objective baseline assessment of auditory and vestibular function should be made and repeated at regular intervals. By the time the patient notices abnormalities, damage is likely to be severe.

Table 5.7 Antibiotic levels and toxicity

Drug	Satisfactory levels (mg/litre) Trough	Peak
Gentamicin	< 2	10–12
Tobramycin	< 2	10–12
Netilmicin	< 2	10–12
Amikacin	< 5	20–30
Vancomycin	< 5	20–30
Chloramphenicol		50
Flucytosine		80

Bactericidal blood levels

A method of monitoring the effectiveness of therapy is to see how well the antibiotic in the blood at times of trough and peak concentration kills the infecting organism. This approach is most often used in cases of endocarditis.

Resistance to antimicrobial agents

Antimicrobial agents work by disrupting some vital microbial structure or function, including cell wall or membrane, or the synthesis of DNA, RNA or protein. First, they have to reach their target; secondly, that target has to be susceptible. If the agent cannot reach its target or if the target does not exist or is not susceptible, the organisms will be resistant.

The aminoglycosides are transported into the cell by oxidative mechanisms. These mechanisms do not exist in anaerobic species which are, therefore, resistant to aminoglycosides. Nitroimidazoles are reduced within bacteria to lethal metabolites; most aerobic species lack the reductase systems necessary for this, and are therefore resistant to nitroimidazoles.

Enzymatic destruction of antimicrobial agents is a common means of resistance. Beta lactamase enzymes inactivate penicillins and cephalosporins. Gram-positive species, such as staphylococci, secrete the beta lactamases into the immediate environment. The beta lactamases of Gram-negative species work within the bacterial cell wall. Aminoglycosides and chloramphenicol can be destroyed within the cell by acetyl transferases, adenylyl transferases or phosphorylating enzymes. The bacterial cell wall itself may present a barrier to antimicrobial agents. Alteration of cell wall penicillin-binding proteins renders organisms resistant to penicillins even in the absence of beta lactamases. Within a bacterial population there may be a few organisms that are resistant. When exposed to the antimicrobial agent, only resistant strains survive and grow. Resistance appears to emerge rapidly, but all that has happened is the selection of pre-existing resistance, as occurs with rifampicin and fusidic acid.

Alternatively, exposure to an antimicrobial agent may induce a genetic mutation resulting in resistance. For aminoglycosides this may be expressed as an alteration in the structure of the target ribosome. This gives immediate or single step high level resistance.

From this is easy to see how the inappropriate or inadequate use of antimicrobial agents can cause bacterial resistance. More important, however, is the capacity of bacteria to transfer DNA coding for such resistance to organisms that have never been exposed to the antibiotic. In this way resistance to many antimicrobial agents can be transferred in a single step.

Genetic transfer of resistance

The portions of DNA coding for resistance can be carried either on the single bacterial chromosome or on smaller, extra-chromosomal, circular DNA elements called plasmids. Resistance (R) plasmids may code for up to nine different agents.

This genetic information may be transferred between bacteria by three processes: transformation, transduction and conjugation.

Transformation is the simplest process. It involves the uptake of free DNA by bacteria.

Conjugation involves the transfer of chromosomal or plasmid DNA from a donor strain to a recipient via a special surface appendage known as a sex pilus. It is the main means of genetic transfer among Gram-negative species.

Transduction depends on bacteriophage – viruses that infect bacteria. Although most bacteriophage lyse bacteria when they attack them, some simply become integrated with the host bacterial genome without causing any apparent damage. When the virus eventually replicates, it may carry away part of the bacterial genome coding for antibiotic resistance. Transduction seems to be an important means of transfer of resistance among staphylococci.

Genetic transfer of resistance effectively speeds up the process by which clinically significant resistance spreads. These processes occur particularly in sites such as the gastro-intestinal and upper respiratory tracts which also provide ideal conditions for the transfer of resistance between commensal and pathogenic organisms.

Further reading

Garrod LP, Lambert HP, O'Grady F. *Antibiotic and Chemotherapy*, 1981; fifth edition, Churchill Livingstone, Edinburgh.
Proceedings of the Second ICI/Stuart Workshop. *Infect Control* 1986; 7, suppl. 2.

6

Wound healing

The healing of wounds is a fundamental characteristic of all living matter –
indeed, life on earth would rapidly be extinguished if it were not so. The
processes of healing have been most extensively investigated in mammals,
and it is these which will be described here, but first the word 'wound' must
be defined. It is easy to narrow the definition to mean a deliberate surgical
wound or an incised or lacerated traumatic wound. The same principles of
healing apply, however, whenever there has been death or disruption of
tissues – a simple fracture, an infarct of an internal organ, ischaemic
gangrene of an extremity, an abscess or an ulcer of skin or mucous
membrane.

The sequence of wound healing is, first, the isolation of the wound from
the rest of the body, then the invasion of what is now recognized to be alien
by neutrophils and macrophages, the removal of dead tissue (and sometimes
bacteria), the ingrowth of new blood vessels and new fibroblasts, the production of collagen and ground substance by the fibroblasts, the replacement of
integument if it has been lost and, finally, the long process of maturation. In
many species maturation reproduces the anatomy and function of the
wounded part, but in mammals this ability appears to be confined to the
liver; after partial hepatectomy there is progressive regeneration of liver cells
and architecture.

Processes of isolation of the wound

Isolation of the wound starts immediately. Small blood vessels are sealed by
platelet aggregations and by coagulated blood; large vessels are sealed by
contraction of their muscular walls followed by coagulation of the blood
within them. In surgical and many traumatic wounds this is helped by the
application of ligatures or coagulating diathermy. The end result, within a
few minutes, is the total isolation of the wound from the rest of the body.
The blood clot within the wound, no less than the dead cells and bacteria, is
alien and must be removed.

Invasion of the wound by leucocytes

The processes of inflammation have been studied for a century, even since
Metchnikoff first showed phagocytosis in amoebae, but many of the trigger
mechanisms are still under investigation. The first event, mediated by kinins

liberated from platelets, is capillary dilatation and stasis, followed by margination and attachment of monocytes and neutrophils along the endothelial walls and their emigration through gaps between the endothelial cells. This chemotaxis is stimulated mainly by activated components of complement, notably C_{3a}. The neutrophils are important not only for phagocytosis but also because their disintegration within the wound releases proteolytic enzymes and prostaglandins which provide the stimulus for the continuation of the inflammatory reaction. Neutrophils do, however, also release highly toxic oxygen radicals which are capable of inflicting damage on the tissues.[1] A key role is played by platelets, both in sealing severed blood vessels and in releasing chemotactic chemicals which attract neutrophils and blood monocytes to the wound.

Blood monocytes and tissue macrophages are activated by lymphokines secreted by lymphocytes, and they are the main scavengers of dead tissue. They also secrete interleukin I ('endogenous pyrogen') and an angiogenesis factor which initiates the budding of endothelial cells from capillaries and their invasion of the wound. Both neutrophils and macrophages are capable of phagocytosis of particles opsonized by plasma fibronectin and activated complement in a relatively anoxic and acidotic environment, but totally anoxic conditions abolish the superoxide-peroxide reaction within phagosomes and thereby reduce the efficiency of intracellular digestion. Hunt and his co-workers showed a gradient of available oxygen from the zero level in the necrotic tissue in the centre of a healing wound to the normal level in arterial blood in the surrounding undamaged tissue.[2] Macrophages, the key cells in the healing sequence, are inactivated in the presence of a Po_2 of less than 30 mmHg, and there appears to be a linear relationship between oxygen availability and the efficiency of healing. It follows that hypovolaemia, anoxia and local ischaemia are potent inhibitors of healing and that the correction of all these defects must be a first priority.

Tetrachlorodecaoxygen anion complex (TCDO) is a novel chemically-stable water-soluble compound containing oxygen in a chlorite matrix. When TCDO is complexed with haem moieties it releases molecular oxygen which stimulates macrophages to perform their dual functions of phagocytosis and fibroplasia. In a multicentre double-blind random control trial in Hannover, Stahl and his colleagues reported that twice-daily application of 5 ml of a solution of TCDO (Oxoferin) in 137 patients had a significantly greater effect on the healing of ulcers – particularly those associated with venous insufficiency – than normal saline dressings in a control group of 134 patients.[3] The beneficial effect was noted not only on the cleansing of the ulcers, but also on the progress of granulations and on epithelialization. TCDO-treated ulcers healed more than twice as fast as those treated with saline.

Collagen

Macrophages secrete a fibroblast-stimulating substance and, in the presence of this and of the growth factor released by dead platelets, fibroblasts begin to invade the wound within 24 hours. They manufacture tropocollagen and the proteoglycans of ground substance within the cells. The production of tropocollagen requires the hydroxylation of proline and lysine, which is dependent on a supply of ferrous iron, a reducing substance such as ascorbic acid, alpha ketoglutarate and oxygen. Both tropocollagen and ground substance are extruded, and they form the scaffolding on which the ultimate repair is effected. Tropocollagen is converted to insoluble collagen, but the fibres are arranged randomly and confer no strength to the wound for many days. Remodelling of the arrangement of the collagen fibres, and the conversion of some of them to elastic fibres, continues for several months, and this is accompanied by contraction of the scar tissue.

Infection and wound healing

Only two types of cell are essential to the initiation of the healing process – platelets and macrophages. When, however, a wound is contaminated by bacteria a new factor emerges: the bacteria themselves, and dead neutrophils, release proteolytic enzymes (including collagenases) which attack and digest not only the new collagen being laid down by fibroblasts, but also the old undamaged collagen. If this bacterial digestion goes far enough from the sutured wound edges, the tissues lose the power to hold the sutures, which consequently tear out. Apart from technical mismanagement, this is the only remaining cause of a burst abdomen now that the principle is universally accepted of using durable suture material placed at least 1 cm away from the cut edges.

Healing cannot take place until all bacteria have been eliminated by the humoral and cellular host defences, and it is in this connection that neturophils play such an important part. Whereas an uninfected wound can heal normally in totally neutropenic animals, an infected wound cannot.

Contraction of the healed wound

The process of remodelling of the arrangement of collagen fibres along the lines of stress involves absorption of errant fibres and reinforcement of those that lie in the right direction. The result is a gradual contraction of the scar, a process which goes on for months. Malt and his co-workers investigated the behaviour of dermal wounds produced by burning and freezing.[4] They found that the maturation of a burn wound in rats reduced its area to one third after 21 days, whereas freeze burns did not contract. They postulated that this was because the architecture of the collagen fibres was preserved in the freeze burns and that the new collagen had a framework already present.

Restoration of integument

If a wound involves loss or incision of skin or mucosa, healing is accompanied by replacement of the integument, by proliferation of cells from surviving glands in the depths of the wound, by ingrowth from the edges, or by the attachment of autologous skin placed there by a surgeon. The forces which direct new integument to align itself on the surface of the wound are ill-understood, as is the nature of the growth factors involved. Infection, particularly by haemolytic streptococci, completely inhibits epithelialization.

Conclusion

The intricate processes of repair and regeneration are only now being explained. Infection and anoxia are the chief inhibitors of rapid healing, and there is as yet no certain way of assisting the healing process apart from the prophylaxis and treatment of infection and the avoidance or correction of anoxia.

References

1. Shandall AA, Williams GT, Hallett MB, Young HL. Colonic healing: a role for polymorphonuclear leucocytes and oxygen radical production. *Brit J Surg* 1986; **73**:225–28.
2. Hunt TK (ed). *Wound Healing and Wound Infection. Theory and Surgical Practice*. New York, Appleton-Century-Crofts, 1980.
3. Hinz J, Hautzinger H, Stahl KW. Rationale for and results from a randomised, double-blind trial of tetrachlorodecaoxygen anion complex in wound healing. *Lancet* 1986; 1:825–28.
4. Li AKC, Ehrlich HP, Trelstad RL, Koroly MJ, Schattenkerk ME, Malt RA. Differences in healing of skin wounds caused by burn and freeze injuries. *Ann Surg* 1980; **191**:244–48.

Part II

The Metabolic and Haemodynamic
Consequences of Sepsis

7

Metabolic and haemodynamic consequences of sepsis

There is some confusion about the use of the word 'sepsis'. Throughout most of the world it is synonymous with generalized infection with or without microbiologically confirmed bacteraemia, whereas in Britain it is often used merely to indicate the presence of pus. I prefer the former interpretation, and it is in this sense that I now use the word sepsis.

We have discussed local and systemic defences against infection in Chapter 4. It is when these defences are overwhelmed by virulent bacteria in large numbers that sepsis arises and patients are exposed to the risks of metabolic derangement and multiple organ failure. A progression is usually observed in these sick patients. The first manifestation is pulmonary failure resulting in adult respiratory distress syndrome; failure of other organs follows and the sequence is often liver, gastric mucosa and kidneys. Cerebral failure and diffuse intravascular coagulation resulting in bleeding are common accompaniments. I propose to discuss these abnormalities under separate headings, recognizing, however, that they interact and that the care of a severely septic patient demands an assessment of all organ systems.

Metabolic derangements associated with sepsis

The metabolic response to sepsis involves glucose first. Hyperglycaemia and insulin resistance are associated with increased serum levels of lactate and pyruvate. Fat metabolism is affected, and the level of plasma triglycerides increases. Finally, amino acids are mobilized from muscles and are used as fuel. The negative nitrogen balance, which is a constant accompaniment of sepsis, reflects both increased catabolism and decreased synthesis. The plasma levels of the aromatic amino acids phenylalanine and tyrosine and the sulphur-containing amino acids taurine, cystine and methionine are elevated;[1] one of the markers of the severity of sepsis is the plasma level of proline which rises with increased severity.

From the practical point of view the importance of the metabolic derangements in sepsis is that these patients rapidly lose weight and that much of this loss is in lean body mass. Plasma albumin concentration falls precipitately; this reduces plasma colloid osmotic pressure and contributes to fluid sequestration in the interstitial spaces. The place of intravenous nutritional support by glucose, fat and amino acids in the treatment of septic patients is still controversial. Overinfusion of glucose leads not to increased oxidation but to conversion of the glucose into fat which is deposited in the liver and elsewhere. Exogenous fat is well tolerated. Up to 1600 KCal (6.7 MJ) per day in a 70 kg adult can be given in the form of glucose; greater metabolic requirements dictate the addition of fat emulsions, but there is scant evidence that amino acid solutions are used for anything other than fuel.[2] If the patient recovers from sepsis, his convalescence is speeded by adequate nutritional intake.

Adult respiratory distress syndrome

'Respiratory failure is present in a subject at rest, breathing air, at sea level, if, because of impaired respiratory function, the arterial blood Po_2 is below 60 mmHg or the Pco_2 is above 49 mmHg'.[3] The function of the lungs is to expose venous blood to air, so that carbon dioxide can diffuse out and oxygen can diffuse in through the alveolar-capillary walls. Failure of this function can therefore be caused by paralysis of the muscles of respiration, by functional or organic obstruction of the major airways, by failure of the right heart to deliver – or the left heart to retrieve – blood, by shunting of venous blood from pulmonary arterioles to venules without passing through shut capillaries, or by changes in the alveolar-capillary interface sufficient to prevent gaseous exchanges.

The term 'adult respiratory distress syndrome', synonymous with 'shock lung', is used to denote the last two of these mechanisms of failure. The most common cause is sepsis, but the condition is also found in other conditions:

- severe pancreatitis
- lung contusion by blast injury or direct trauma
- lung damage by inhalation of smoke or other toxic fumes
- fat embolism
- aspiration of gastric contents.

Adult respiratory distress syndrome must be distinguished from pulmonary oedema as a result of fluid overload and from the syndrome of hypovolaemic or cardiogenic shock.

What causes pulmonary failure in septic patients?

Detailed histological examination of the lungs of 44 patients who died with respiratory failure caused by the adult respiratory distress syndrome showed that thrombi in small pulmonary vessels were more often found than in the lungs of 31 control patients.[4] There seems no doubt that the cross-sectional area of the pulmonary vasculature is reduced: this is reflected in the raised pulmonary artery pressure which is a universal accompaniment of the syndrome.[5] Whether this is a result of thrombo-embolism or of leakage of fluid through damaged capillaries into the interstitial space is conjectural, but there is evidence that fluid sequestration into the third space plays an important role, and that the capillary damage is mediated by circulating toxins associated with sepsis.[6]

The concept of capillary leakage is, however, an oversimplification, and serial lung biopsies have shown that there is a rapid replacement of alveolar epithelium by proliferating type II cuboidal cells, capillary obliteration and interstitial inflammation resulting in fibrosis. In an extensive review Rinaldo and Rogers discussed the pathogenesis of pulmonary endothelial injury and the role of complement, neutrophils and proteases.[7] Activated complement (C5a) induces neutrophil aggregation in pulmonary capillaries; these neutrophils then break up, releasing superoxide and proteases in sufficient quantities to neutralize alpha-1-antitrypsin. The proteases attack and destroy alveolar epithelium and interstitial tissues. The role of complement activation and neutrophil disintegration is disputed by other workers, who lay stress on the aggregration of platelets causing intravascular coagulation and release of toxic fibrin degradation products.[8]

There is also evidence of increasing shunting of venous blood to the pulmonary veins without passing through the capillaries, and of cellular swelling. It has been suggested that plasma fibronectin (opsonic protein) deficiency reduces the capacity of the reticulo-endothelial system to clear particulate matter from the circulation.[9] The enhancement of reticulo-endothelial function by drugs such as muramyl dipeptide, the replacement of fibronectin by infusion of fresh frozen plasma, and the correction of cellular swelling by hypertonic mannitol infusion are all therapeutic possibilities which have not yet been extensively investigated clinically.

Clinical features of adult respiratory distress syndrome

The patient is hyperpnoeic and the arterial Po_2 is below 60 mmHg. He is obviously ill and mentally confused. Chest X-rays show a 'snow storm' appearance which is consistent with pulmonary oedema, and there is increased resistance to ventilation. Pulmonary infection is always a risk, either from an endogenous source by the organisms causing the sepsis or from exogenous sources including endotracheal tubes and ventilation equipment.

Treatment

The treatment of a patient with respiratory failure secondary to sepsis requires consideration of the following: treatment of sepsis by operation and antibiotics, maintenance of circulating blood volume, correction of hypoxaemia, cardiac support, and possibly the use of steroids.

Treatment of sepsis

In general surgical practice most sepsis arises from abdominal disease or the complications of abdominal surgery. Clinical examination, ultrasonography and computerized tomography play important roles in the location of intra-abdominal abscesses. These are very ill patients, but we should remember the axiom that such patients are too ill *not* to be operated on, and the removal of an infected focus or the drainage of an abscess in the abdomen is probably the most important aspect of treatment. At the same time, antibiotics appropriate to the anticipated bacteria must be prescribed.

Maintenance of blood volume

Sequestration of fluid, electrolytes and colloids in the third space results in hypovolaemia and aggravates the poor tissue oxygenation caused by respiratory failure. The difficulty is that any solution administered intravenously to these patients results in further extravasation into the lungs and elsewhere, and this occurs whether the solution is of colloids, colloids plus crystalloids, or crystalloids alone. It is certain that infusion of glucose alone is useless and possibly harmful.

Shoemaker and Hauser put forward arguments in favour of colloid infusions,[10] and they showed that in dogs 500 ml of colloid solution or blood were more effective in restoring haemodynamics and oxygen transport than 1000 ml of Ringer lactate solution. The alternative view is that infusion of solutions containing albumin results in further extravasation of the protein into the interstitial tissue and that this is harmful.[11] Whichever fluid is used (and in the absence of convincing clinical work I shall continue to prefer Ringer lactate solution), the amount infused should be monitored by serial estimations of the central venous – or preferably the pulmonary capillary wedge – pressure, the response of these pressures to rapid infusion, and by aiming at a haematocrit of 35 per cent which allows optimal oxygen delivery because of reduced whole blood viscosity.

Correction of hypoxaemia

When arterial hypoxia cannot be corrected by administration of oxygen-enriched air by face mask, the treatment of respiratory failure by mechanical ventilation with positive end-expiratory pressure, introduced by Ashbaugh in 1967,[12] is widely practised. There are several complications of the technique, including pneumothorax, oxygen toxicity if the inspired air contains more than 30 per cent of oxygen, and exogenous bronchopulmonary infection. Nevertheless, it is likely that mechanical ventilation has reduced the case fatality rate in septic shock. In all cases, care must be taken to remove secretions and humidify the inspired oxygen-rich air in order to prevent major airways obstruction.

There has been considerable interest among anaesthetists in the technique of high frequency ventilation, but a controlled clinical trial failed to show any advantage over normal controlled mechanical ventilation in patients with adult respiratory distress syndrome.[13]

Cardiac support

Many patients with respiratory failure show signs of cardiac failure with or without arrhythmias. Treatment with digoxin, dopamine, adrenaline and isoproterenol must be considered in all cases.

Steroids

It has been claimed that massive intravenous doses of methyl prednisolone are beneficial, possibly because of the membrane-stabilizing effect of the drug. Controlled clinical trials have, however, failed to substantiate the benefits shown in experimental work.[14]

Failure of other organ systems

Hepatic dysfunction is common in association with sepsis, and this may progress to obvious clinical jaundice with a biochemical profile of cholestasis. Brain failure is an early sign of sepsis and progresses from withdrawal of interest in the surroundings to confusion, stupor and coma. It is often aggravated by the sedative drugs which are necessary for the comfort of any patient undergoing continous invasive monitoring and treatment.

There is no specific treatment for either liver failure or brain failure, and the clinical results of steroid administration are disappointing.

Renal failure is common in septic patients, and its severity varies from oliguria (or occasionally polyuria) with a rise in the levels of urea and creatinine in the blood, to acute tubular necrosis and anuria. Although haemodialysis or peritoneal dialysis allows time for the kidneys to recover, the syndrome is so often complicated by failure of other organ systems that severe renal failure has a bad prognosis; no more than half these patients survive. Two aspects of treatment require special consideration: first, over-infusion of fluid must be avoided and, secondly, glucose must be given to counteract hyperkalaemia.

Gastro-intestinal failure usually shows itself in the form of haematemesis from gastric erosions. Workers in Creteil showed that gastric erosions can always be demonstrated endoscopically in septic patients.[15] Intravenous cimetidine or ranitidine, coupled with monitoring of gastric pH and titration towards neutrality by oral administration of alkalis, reduce the incidence of gastric bleeding. Groll and his colleagues studied patients in a general intensive care unit.[16] Of 531 eligible patients, 221 were randomized to receive intravenous cimetidine 300 mg 6-hourly (n = 114) or placebo (n = 107). There were six clinical bleeding episodes in the cimetidine group compared with 11 in the control group (P = 0.16). There is a large Type II error in concluding that cimetidine was no better than placebo.

Two uncommon, but desperately serious, complications of severe sepsis are acalculous gangrenous cholecystitis and intestinal gangrene in the absence of vascular occlusion. Both these events are more frequently diagnosed *post mortem* than during life.

A terminal event in some patients with severe sepsis and multiple organ system failure is internal bleeding resulting from diffuse intravascular coagulation and the depletion of cellular and humoral components of the clotting system. One should always be on the watch for dangerous depletion, particularly of platelets and fibrinogen, and be prepared to infuse these intravenously.

Conclusions

Severe sepsis, coupled sometimes with the treatment required to overcome the problems that it raises, can result in failure of nearly all the organ systems of the body. This failure is caused by circulating toxins which damage capillary endothelium, resulting in leakage of fluid and protein into the interstitial spaces. Activated complement causes aggregation and disintegration of neutrophils and the release of toxic hydrogen/oxygen radicals and proteases. Platelet aggregates obstruct arterioles and capillaries, and tissue anoxia results from a combination of all these factors. Increased metabolic demands rapidly deplete liver stores of glycogen, and fat and muscle protein are mobilized to provide fuel. The utilization of glucose is inefficient, and insulin resistance is usual. Surgical therapeutic prowess falls far short of ideal, and nearly half of all seriously septic patients die despite (and occasionally because of) the best supportive treatment that can be offered.

References

1. Freund HR, Ryan JA, Fischer JE. Amino acid derangements in patients with sepsis: treatment with branched chain amino acid rich infusions. *Ann Surg* 1978; **188**:423–30.
2. MacFie J. Towards cheaper intravenous nutrition. *Br Med J* 1986; **292**:107–10.
3. Campbell EJM. Respiratory failure. *Br Med J* 1965; **i**:1451–60.
4. Davis HA, Pollak EW. Adult respiratory distress syndrome in postoperative patients: study of pulmonary pathology in shock lung with prophylactic and therapeutic implications. *Amer Surg* 1975; **41**:391–97.
5. Anonymous. Pulmonary hypertension in acute respiratory failure. *Lancet* 1977; **ii**:283–84.
6. Clowes GHA, Farrington GH, Zuschneid W, Cossette GR, Saravis C. Circulating factors in the etiology of pulmonary insufficiency and right heart failure accompanying severe sepsis (peritonitis). *Ann Surg* 1970; **171**:663–78.
7. Rinaldo JE, Rogers RM. Adult respiratory distress syndrome. Changing concepts of lung injury and repair. *New Engl. J Med* 1982; **306**:900–909.
8. Bell RC, Coalson JJ, Smith JD, Johanson WG. Multiple organ system failure and infection in adult respiratory distress syndrome. *Ann Intern Med* 1983; **99**:293–98.
9. Niehaus G, Schumacker PT, Saba TM. Reticuloendothelial clearance of blood-borne particulates in sheep: relevance of lung microembolization and vascular injury. *Ann Surg* 1980; **191**:479–82.
10. Shoemaker WC, Hauser CJ. Critique of crystalloid versus colloid therapy in shock and shock lung. *Crit Care Med* 1979: **7**:117–24.
11. Deysine M, Stein S. Albumin shifts across the extracellular space secondary to experimental infections. *Surg Gynecol Obstet* 1980; **151**:617–19.
12. Ashbaugh DG, Bigelow DB, Petty TL, Levine BE. Acute respiratory distress in adults. *Lancet* 1967; **ii**:319–23.
13. Carlon GC, Howland WS, Ray C *et al.* High frequency-jet ventilation. A prospective randomized evaluation. *Chest* 1983; **84**:551–59.
14. Lucas CE, Ledgerwood AM. Pulmonary response of massive steroids in seriously injured patients. *Ann Surg* 1981; **194**:256–61.
15. Le Gall JR, Mignon FC, Rapin M, Redjemi M, Harari A, Bader JP, Soussy CJ. Acute gastroduodenal lesions related to severe sepsis. *Surg Gynecol Obstet* 1976; **142**:377–80.
16. Groll A, Simon JB, Wigle RD, Taguchi K, Todd RJ, Depew WT. Cimetidine prophylaxis for gastrointestinal bleeding in an intensive care unit. *Gut* 1986; **27**:135–40.

8

Assessment of severity of sepsis

The outcome of an infective illness depends on the balance between the resistance of the host on the one hand, and the number and virulence of the invading bacteria on the other. Unless an objective assessment of both these factors is made, there is no way of comparing the results of one therapeutic regimen with another using historical, non-random contemporary or randomized controls, nor can the results from one unit be compared with those from another.

Most of the sepsis which concerns general surgeons originates in the abdomen and Dawson was one of the first surgeons to point out that the outcome of peritonitis depends on the age of the patient and the cause of the peritonitis.[1] Since the early 1960s there have been several attempts to quantify the risk of death in patients with sepsis and other serious illnesses. These scores have evolved in the setting of surgical intensive care units, and their origins can be traced back to 1974 when Baker and his colleagues in Baltimore published their Injury Severity Score (the sum of the squares of values from 0 to 5 for the severity of each of three most severely injured parts),[2] and Cullen and his colleagues in Boston published the Therapeutic Intervention Scoring System (57 items graded from 1 for simple monitoring to 4 for complex treatments like haemodialysis).[3]

The scoring system which I have adopted was first put forward by Knaus and his colleagues in 1981[4] and was simplified in 1984.[5] Tables 8.1 and 8.2 are taken from the paper from Ledingham's unit and are reproduced by permission of the Editor of the British Medical Journal.[6] The Glasgow coma scale is displayed in Table 8.3.

The importance of Knaus's score which he calls the Acute Physiology and Chronic Health Evaluation (APACHE) is that it allows comparisons of the results of treatment within a unit and between one unit and another. Knaus and his colleagues surveyed 795 consecutive admissions to intensive care units in five hospitals in the United States. They found that the APACHE score accurately predicted the death rates, ranging from 5 per cent for a score less than 5, 6 per cent for scores of 6–10, 10 per cent for scores of 10–15, 20 per cent for scores of 16–20, 30 per cent for scores of 21–25, 50 per cent for scores of 26–30, 60 per cent for scores of 31–35 and 75 per cent for scores of over 36.[7] They further validated the score by an international comparison of the results in five United States hospitals with those in seven French hospitals.[8]

Meakins and others used the APACHE score with weightings for increasing age[9] and, subsequently,[10] also for malnutrition to define a Surgical Infection

Table 8.1 Sickness scores: values for individual variables

	4	3	2	1	Score 0	1	2	3	4
Core temperature (°C)	≥41	39–40.9	—	38.5–38.9	36–38.4	34–35.9	32–33.9	30–31.9	≤29.9
Mean blood pressure (mmHg)*	≥160	130–159	110–129	—	70–109	—	50–69	—	≤49
Heart rate/min	≥180	140–179	110–139	—	70–109	—	55–69	40–54	≤39
Respiratory rate/min	≥50	35–49	—	25–34	12–24	10–11	6–9	—	≤5
% inspired O_2/Pao_2(kPa)	≥5.0	4.0–4.99	2.1–3.99	—	<2.09	—	—	—	—
Arterial pH	≥7.7	7.6–7.69	—	7.5–7.59	7.33–7.49	—	7.25–7.32	7.15–7.24	≤7.15
Creatinine (μmol/litre)†	≥600	300–599	180–299	130–179	50–129	—	≤49	—	—
Sodium (mmol/litre)	≥180	160–179	155–159	150–154	130–149	—	120–129	111–119	≤110
Potassium (mmol/litre)	≥7.0	6.0–6.9	—	5.5–5.9	3.5–5.4	3.0–3.4	2.5–2.9	—	<2.5
Haemoglobin (g/dl)	≥18.0	—	15.0–17.9	14.0–14.9	9.0–13.9	—	6.1–8.9	—	≤6.0
White cell count (×10^9/litre)	≥40.0	—	20.0–39.9	15.0–19.9	3.0–14.9	—	1.0–2.9	—	<1.0
Glasgow coma scale	Score as 15 minus actual score								

*Mean arterial pressure (mmHg) = (2 diastolic + systolic)/3
†If acute renal failure has occurred, double score
Conversion: SI to traditional units – Pao_2: 1 kPa = 7.5 mmHg. Creatinine: 1 μmol/litre = 0.01 mg/100 ml. Sodium: 1 mmol/litre = 1 mEq/litre.
Potassium: 1 mmol/litre = 1 mEq/litre.
Reprinted from: Bion JF et al. Br Med J 1985; **291**:433 by permission of the publisher.

Table 8.2 Scores for age and chronic disease

Age (years)	≤44	45–54	55–64	65–74	≥75
Score	0	2	3	5	6

Chronic disease score
If chronic disease history is positive:
elective postoperative patients score 2
emergency postoperative or medical patients score 5

Chronic disease category
1 Disease (a) must have been evident before this hospital admission; (b) must be of sufficient severity to prevent independent self care
   This category includes chronic dialysis, documented cirrhosis, or portal hypertension, and disease of other systems of severity which will generally confine patient to the house
2 Immunosuppression: patients receiving chemotherapy, radiation, long-term low-dose steroids, or short-term high-dose steroids; or malignant or other disease which is sufficiently advanced to impair resistance to infection

Reprinted from: Bion JF *et al. Br Med J* 1985; **291**:433 by permission of the publisher.

Table 8.3 Glasgow coma scale

Best verbal response		Best motor response		Eye opening	
None	1	None	1	None	1
Incomprehensible	2	Extending	2	To pain	2
Inappropriate	3	Abnormal flexion	3	To speech	3
Confused	4	Flexion to pain	4	Spontaneous	4
Orientated	5	Localizing pain	5		
		Obeying commands	6		

Stratification System for intra-abdominal infections, taking account of the varying prognoses of infections originating in the stomach and duodenum (group I), small intestine (group II), large intestine (group III), from postoperative complications (group IV) and appendix (group VII). They pointed out that the reported mortality rate from peritonitis in some therapeutic trials of antibiotics in 'serious intra-abdominal infections' has been as low as 3.5 per cent, whereas audits of consecutive cases often show mortality rates in excess of 30 per cent. It is clear that stratification for risk must be made in all therapeutic trials.

Pre-operative assessment of the chances of surviving a major operation

Generations of surgeons have made subjective assessments of the risks of patients dying after operations, but there have been few attempts to quantify these risks. The American Society of Anesthesiologists classified physical

Table 8.4 ASA (American Society of Anesthesiologists) classification of physical status

Class 1   The patient has no organic, physiological, biochemical, or psychiatric disturbance. The pathological process for which operation is to be performed is localized and does not entail a systemic disturbance. Examples: a fit patient with an inguinal hernia; fibroid uterus in an otherwise healthy woman.

Class 2   Mild to moderate systemic disturbance caused either by the condition to be treated surgically or by other pathophysiological processes. Examples: non- or only slightly limiting organic heart disease, mild diabetes, essential hypertension, or anaemia. Some might choose to list the extremes of age here, either the neonate or the octogenerian, even though no discernible systemic disease is present. Extreme obesity and chronic bronchitis may be included in this category.

Class 3   Severe systemic disturbance or disease from whatever cause, even though it may not be possible to define the degree of disability with finality. Examples: severely limiting organic heart disease; severe diabetes with vascular complications; moderate to severe degrees of pulmonary insufficiency; angina pectoris or healed myocardial infarction.

Class 4   Severe systemic disorders that are already life threatening, not always correctable by operation. Examples: patients with organic heart disease showing marked signs of cardiac insufficiency, persistent angina, or active myocarditis; advanced degrees of pulmonary, hepatic, renal or endocrine insufficiency.

Class 5   The moribund patient who has little chance of survival but is submitted to operation in desperation. Examples: the burst abdominal aneurysm with profound shock; major cerebral trauma with rapidly increasing intracranial pressure; massive pulmonary embolus. Most of these patients require operation as a resuscitative measure with little if any anesthesia.

status into four classes (Table 8.4), and I have evolved a score system which fits into my computerized audit scheme (Table 8.5). It allows a score of 0 to 10 + , and I have validated it in a consecutive series of 1568 patients undergoing emergency or elective abdominal operations (Table 8.6). Only one patient died within 30 days of operation (from anastomotic failure) of the 713 whose pre-operative scores were 0, compared with 59 of the 92 patients whose scores were 9 or more (64 per cent). The cut-off point seems to be a score of 6. Of 1259 patients who scored 5 or less, 11 died (0.9 per cent), whereas 137 of the 309 (44.3 per cent) of those with a score of 6 or more died.

Other authors have studied anthropometric, biochemical and immunological defects in attempts to define the likely outcome of major operations. The anthropometric measurements are indices of malnutrition, and they include estimation of weight loss (a reduction from the patient's normal weight by 20 per cent, or a rapid reduction by 10 per cent), body mass index (weight in kg divided by height in metres squared) below the third percentile

Table 8.5 Assessment of Fitness Score (Pollock)

The **Assessment of Fitness Score** is constructed by totalling scores for age, chronic diseases and acute (presenting) disease. It is graded 0–10.

Score
1 each	cardiac symptoms controlled by treatment
	short of breath on climbing stairs
	morning cough
	previous stroke
	Hb < 10 g/dl
	albumin 30–35 g/litre
	urea 10–19 mmol/litre
	steroids
	diabetes
2 each	age 70–79 years
	cardiac symptoms not controlled by treatment
	short of breath on walking
	persistent cough with sputum
	confusion
3 each	clinical jaundice
	albumin < 30 g/litre
	loss of 10% weight in 1 month
	urea 20 + mmol/litre
	short of breath at rest
	myocardial infarct within 6 months
4 each	age 80 + years
	palliative operation for cancer
	intestinal obstruction
	perforations, pancreatitis and intraperitoneal abscess (not including perforated appendix)
4 each	haemorrhage or anaemia requiring transfusion
	cytotoxics

Example
A 76-year-old man with a history of controlled angina and mild chronic bronchitis who presents with intestinal obstruction and is operated on for an obstructing carcinoma with liver metastases would score 2 (age) + 1 (heart) + 1 (respiratory) + 4 (obstruction) + 4 (palliative operation) – total 12, coded on computer as 0.

of published standards for age and sex, triceps skinfold thickness, midarm circumference and the derived midarm muscle circumference, and hand-grip strength. Critical biochemical values are < 33 g/litre for albumin, < 1.5 g/litre for transferrin and < 0.12 g/litre for pre-albumin.

Table 8.6 Validation of assessment of fitness score

Score	Number of patients	Number of deaths (%)
0	713	1 (0.1)
1	76	0 (0)
2	151	2 (1.3)
3	98	0 (0)
4	139	5 (3.6)
5	82	3 (3.7)
6	74	21 (28.4)
7	70	28 (40.0)
8	73	29 (39.7)
9	66	43 (65.2)
10 +	26	16 (61.5)
Total	1568	148 (9.4)

Immunological defects are most easily recognized by intradermal injection of four or five recall antigens (mumps, Candida, trichophyton, purified protein derivative of old tuberculin and streptokinase/streptodornase); the diameter of the resulting weal is measured 24 and 48 hours later. People with normal cell-mediated immunity produce a weal greater than 5 mm in diameter in response to two or more antigens, relatively anergic people respond to one antigen, and anergic people respond to none. Anergy or relative anergy is certainly associated with trauma or sepsis, but its importance as a pre-operative predictor of death or complications is controversial. Work in my unit and in Manchester failed to confirm that patients found to be anergic or relatively anergic before elective operations suffered significantly more complications or a higher death rate than normally-reacting patients.[11, 12]

Pettigrew and Hill concluded that careful clinical assessment combined with serum protein measurements (transferrin and pre-albumin being more sensitive than albumin) were more valuable than anthropometric measurements in predicting high-risk patients.[13] They allotted a score of 1 each for bronchitis, smoking, treated hypertension, mild angina, past history of rheumatic fever or tuberculosis, diabetes, high alcohol intake and mild nutritional deficiency. Moderate nutritional deficiency scored 2 and severe deficiency 3, whereas a score of 4 each was allotted to severe obstructive airways disease, current chest infection, recent myocardial infarction, presence of a pacemaker, previous pneumonectomy, jaundice, failure of renal, cardiac or respiratory function, prolonged high-dose steroids, thrombocytopenia, metastatic cancer or myeloma, major sepsis and past history of venous thrombosis or pulmonary embolism. In their system a score of 6 or more indicated a high risk of death or complications.

Conclusions

It is essential in considering trials of the treatment of sepsis to compare like with like, and the stratification of severity of illness and chances of dying allow comparisons within a unit and between one unit and another. The assessment of the risks of complications or death following major operations is made most accurately by careful clinical assessment of patients.

References

1. Dawson JL. A study of some factors affecting the mortality rate in diffuse peritonitis. *Gut* 1963; **4**:368–72.
2. Baker S, O'Neill B, Haddon W, Long WB. The injury severity score: a method for describing patients with multiple injuries and evaluating emergency care. *J Trauma* 1974; **14**:187–96.
3. Cullen DJ, Civetta JM, Briggs BA, Ferrara LC. Therapeutic intervention scoring system: a method for quantitative comparison of patient care. *Crit Care Med* 1974; **2**:57–60.
4. Knaus WA, Zimmerman JE, Wagner DP, Draper EA, Lawrence DE. APACHE – acute physiology and chronic health evaluation: a physiologically based classification system. *Crit Care Med* 1981; **9**:591–603.
5. Knaus WA, Draper EA, Wagner DP, Zimmerman JE. APACHE II: a severity of disease classification system. *Crit Care Med* 1985; **13**:818–29.
6. Bion JF, Edlin SA, Ramsay G, McCabe S, Ledingham I McA. Validation of a prognostic score in critically ill patients undergoing transport. *Br Med J* 1985; **291**:432–34.
7. Knaus WA, Draper EA, Wagner DP, *et al.* Evaluating outcome from intensive care: a preliminary multihospital comparison. *Crit Care Med* 1982; **10**:491–96.
8. Knaus WA, Wagner DP, Loirat P, *et al.* A comparison of intensive care in the USA and France. *Lancet* 1982; **ii**:642–46.
9. Meakins JL, Solomkin JS, Allo MD, Dellinger EP, Howard RJ, Simmons RL. A proposed classification of intra-abdominal infections: stratification of etiology and risk, for future therapeutic trials. *Arch Surg* 1984; **119**:1372–78.
10. Dellinger EP, Wertz MJ, Meakins JL, *et al.* Surgical infection stratification system for intra-abdominal infection. *Arch Surg* 1985; **120**:21–29.
11. Ausobsky JR, Bean P, Proctor J, Pollock AV. Delayed hypersensitivity testing for the prediction of postoperative complications. *Br J Surg* 1982; **69**:346–48.
12. Brown R, Bancewicz J, Hamid J, *et al.* Failure of delayed hypersensitivity skin testing to predict postoperative sepsis and mortality. *Br Med J* 1982; **284**:851–53.
13. Pettigrew RA, Hill GL. Indicators of surgical risk and clinical judgement. *Br J Surg* 1986; **73**:47–51.

Part III

The Evaluation of Prophylactic and Therapeutic Regimens

9

Clinical audit

'The purpose (of audit) is to evaluate the quality of care objectively and systematically with the aim of improvement'.[1]

My medical education took place during the last years of the dogmatic surgeon. Woe betide the junior staff, in those days, when the chief advised a woman with carcinoma of the breast to have a radical mastectomy, if they suggested that other surgeons seemed to be getting good results from simple mastectomy with postoperative radiotherapy. When you did a radical mastectomy you had to take away as much skin as possible, you had to make thin flaps, and you had to clean the axilla so that every nerve, artery and vein was distinguishable. When the flaps sloughed and the patient stayed in hospital for a month or more, this was no more than a reasonable price to pay for curing the cancer. You accepted stiff shoulders, lop-sided chests and swollen arms as natural events, and it was the patient's fault if metastases appeared. The stereotype of the successful surgeon caricatured by writers from Moliére to Gordon was of a man who knew all the answers, whose word was all powerful and whose opinion was accepted without question.

How different things are today! Most of the new generation of surgeons are more conscious of questions than of answers. When such a person conducts a ward round he is not afraid to admit his doubts, he encourages divergent views and he is aware at all times of the possibility of complications and the reasons for them. He is constantly trying to improve his practice.

The philosophy of audit

Sir Karl Popper, probably the most important living philosopher of science, summed up his doctrine in these words: 'If we respect truth, we must search for it by persistently searching for our errors, by indefatigable rational criticism and self-criticism'. Scientists can never prove that a hypothesis is true, only that the alternative hypothesis is untrue. Popper and McIntyre put forward 10 theses for a new ethic of critical evaluation in medicine;[2] these can be summarized as follows:

'Our attitude towards mistakes must change. It is here that ethical reform must begin. For the old attitude leads to the hiding of our mistakes and to forgetting them as fast as we can . . . It is therefore our task to search for our mistakes and to investigate them fully. We must train ourselves to be self critical'.

The essence of audit is evaluation. By whom shall the work of a surgeon be evaluated? First and foremost by the surgeon himself, next by the members of his unit, then by his peers in the same hospital and, finally, by his peers in his own country and in the world.

Many surgical activities have economic, ethical, moral and legal consequences. It is the members of the medical staff of a hospital who are responsible for spending most of the money in that hospital, and we must not be surprised if administrators attempt to audit surgical work in relation to costs. We should not, however, deny or resent the rights of our patients to decide for themselves between conflicting policies. Concerning moral issues, we must realize that when we take the beating heart from a dead person, the community will need assurance that we have established that that person is indeed dead. We must expect the whole country to be concerned about the length of waiting lists in some specialities. From the legal point of view surgeons must avoid, on the one hand, negligence and, on the other hand, trespass – the act of operating on a patient without informing him or her of all the material risks as well as benefits associated with the operation.

What surgeons must ensure is that audit (critical evaluation) is constructive, that it leads to better treatment for sick people, to better use of limited financial resources, to the elimination of diseases and injuries which cause premature death, and to satisfaction within and outside the profession.

The components of audit

Clinical audit is incomplete unless all three aspects – structure, process and outcome – are considered.

Audit of structure

In many ways this is the easiest audit to implement. It asks the question: are the necessary facilities there? On a national scale in the United Kingdom this is one of the questions which the Office of Health Economics tries to answer. Are there enough doctors and nurses? Are there enough beds? Are those beds being efficiently used? Are there enough operating theatres, and what proportion of the time do they stand empty? Is endoscopic, radiological and ultrasound equipment available and efficient? Which hospitals should have computerized tomography and isotope detection equipment?

Audit of process

This is a concept taken from industry and its validation relies on the belief that if one takes the right steps (history, examination, appropriate special tests, appropriate treatment) the outcome is likely to be satisfactory. McColl has been a strong protagonist of process audit, and has established numerical norms for the handling of common surgical conditions.[3] He admits, however, that it is impossible to place a numerical value on many processes, such as surgical judgement. It is difficult to get all the surgeons in a hospital to agree to the numerical evaluation of aspects of process. He gives an example of the scores awarded (to a maximum of 14) for procedures carried out on patients admitted for repair of inguinal hernias at Guy's Hospital in London. They are:

- pre-operative haemoglobin, 3 points
- chest X-ray, 3 points
- electrolytes and urea, 1 point
- blood pressure on admission, 3 points
- urinalysis, 1 point
- weight, 1 point
- rectal examination, 2 points

The patient, however, is far more interested in aspects of assessment which score nothing in this scheme, but which may be fundamental to the outcome of the operation. The score system pays scant attention to the physical examination – was this confined to asking the patient to drop his trousers and inspecting and palpating his groins? How careful a history was taken – was the patient asked if he could walk up a flight of stairs without getting short of breath, whether he had to get up at night to pass urine, and whether he coughed most mornings and what the sputum was like? Had he any bowel trouble? Did the surgeon enquire about the domestic circumstances of the patient? Was he suitable for day-case or overnight-stay repair? Would local or general anaesthesia be more appropriate? Was the patient told what a hernia is, and what the surgeon proposed to do about it? Was the patient given a date and time for the operation, and did this take account of his commitments, both work and leisure?

I have outlined a scheme for the management of a patient with an inguinal hernia which most surgeons would regard as proper. How can you audit it? What numerical value would you place on kindness and courtesy relative to efficient and long-lasting repair of the hernia? This is one of the problems of process auditing.

Audit of outcome

The institute of Medicine in Washington, DC, stated in 1974 that 'The Committee believe strongly that the goal of quality assurance can only be achieved by relating assessments of quality to the measurement of results'.[4]

Ernest Amory Codman was on the staff of Massachusetts General Hospital at the beginning of this century and is chiefly remembered for his advocacy of 'end result analysis'.[5] He wrote that 'comparisons are odious, but comparison is necessary in science. Until we freely make therapeutic comparisons, we cannot claim that a given hospital is efficient, for efficiency implies that the results have been looked into . . . Every hospital should follow every patient it treats long enough to determine whether or not the treatment has been successful, and then to enquire "if not, why not?" with a view to preventing similar failures in the future.'[6]

This is the essence of the audit of outcome, but it is only now that physicians are beginning to overcome their fears of the process. Codman's system was introduced at Massachusetts General Hospital in 1912, but it fell into disuse through neglect (wilful?) by the doctors. The young American College of Surgeons issued criteria for hospital acceptability, which included the collection of data on patient outcome. Only 89 of 692 hospitals with more than 100 beds fulfilled these criteria and the survey was destroyed.[6]

If we are going to audit the outcome of our operations, we must be completely honest in our recording. Our audit must be confidential, so that no one is inhibited from recording the truth for fear of legal action. The recording may be merely in a diary, but nowadays it is more useful to enter data about our patients into a microcomputer, using suitable software and codings. One of the most important questions asked in my computer program is about postoperative complications which are described as 'none', 'minor' and 'major'. There is a code for 'points for discussion' which are divided into diagnostic, operative, postoperative and serious drug toxicity. These are the events which one wishes to recall for repeated consideration by members of the unit. For this purpose a weekly or monthly 'deaths and complications' conference is invaluable.

Comparing like with like in clinical audit

If we are going to learn anything from a system of audit, we must compare our results with those of our own in previous years, and with those of other physicians. We must, however, be careful to compare like with like, and this requirement is best met by systems of scoring the severity of illnesses.

The evolution of scoring systems

Considering the magnificent intellectual achievements of the ancient Greeks and Arabs, of mediaeval Italians and of French and English eighteenth century philosophers, it comes as a shock to realize that it was not until the beginning of the nineteenth century in Paris (and then against a hurricane of criticism) that Charles-Alexandre Louis introduced the 'numerical method' in medicine. In a classical paper on the assessment of the results of blood-letting in fevers, he attached numerical values to evaluation of outcome and concluded that blood-letting seldom did any good.[7]

The systematic establishment of scoring systems, and their validation in prospective studies of consecutive series of patients in centres all over the world, has been a phenomenon of the last half-century, proceeding hand in hand with that most sophisticated form of audit, the random control clinical trial. It is inconceivable that a publication about the results of diagnosis or treatment of any disease will ignore an appropriate scoring system, even if the author goes no further than to divide patients into 'high risk' and 'low risk'.

Conclusion

Not only must audit be honest, not only include all patients who come under our care, but also we must compare like with like, and in auditing the outcome of our patients we must be in a position to say 'a patient of ours has just died or suffered a major complication. What could we have done (or left undone) to avert this, bearing in mind the severity of the patient's illness?'

The purpose of audit is to improve the care of patients, to avoid complacency, to be ready for self-criticism and to educate the next generation of doctors in the discipline of lifelong learning.

References

1. Gruer R, Gordon DS, Gunn AA, Ruckley CV. Audit of surgical audit. *Lancet* 1986; i:23–25.
2. McIntyre N, Popper K. The critical attitude in medicine: the need for a new ethics. *Br Med J* 1983; **287**:1919–23.
3. McColl I. Medical audit in British hospital practice. *Br J Hosp Med* 1979; **22**:485–89.
4. Institute of Medicine. Advancing the Quality of Care. *A policy statement by a Committee of the Institute of Medicine.* National Academy of Sciences, Washington DC, 1974.
5. Codman EA. Report of committee on hospital standardization. *Surg Gynec Obstet* 1916; **22**:119–20.
6. Christoffel T. Medical care evaluation: an old new idea. *J Med Educ* 1976; **51**:83–88.
7. Gaines WJ, Langford HG. Research on the effect of blood-letting in several inflammatory maladies. *Arch Intern Med* 1960; **106**:571–79.

10

Clinical trials

Historical introduction

It was Leonardo da Vinci who claimed that no human investigation could be called true science without passing through mathematical tests. Since then it has been by a strange and tortuous route that the mathematics of probability has become applied to the art and science of surgery.

Lack of knowledge of statistical methods was, however, not the only factor militating against the scientific evaluation of treatments. First, there was the ingrained reverence for authority. Where remedies were few, belief in the physician himself was essential. The transition from arguments based on concepts to those based on scientific empiricism was slow.

Where there was an ignorance of pathology and a paucity of effective cures there could be no comparison of 'better' or 'worse' treatments. It was the evolution of microbiology and cellular pathology which made it possible to start understanding diseases instead of grouping them under general, meaningless headings like fever, decline and dropsy.

The process of the application of mathematical theories to medicine was gradual; Blaise Pascal in the seventeenth century concerned himself with the theories of probability in relation to games of chance, and two centuries later Charles-Alexandre Louis developed the so-called 'numerical method'. But it was not until the late nineteenth and early twentieth century that statistical tests of probability began to evolve.

Sir Ronald Fisher, through his work in agricultural research, developed the exact probability test that bears his name.[1] Karl Pearson worked out the chi-square test in 1890, and Gossett – working at the Guinness brewery and writing under the pseudonym of 'Student' – gave us the 't' test. The word 'random' was not used in a statistical sense until the end of the nineteenth century, and 'randomize' not until 1936. After the Second World War, and mainly in North America, Wilcoxon, Mann, Whitney and others developed ranking tests for data which are not normally distributed.

The application of all this knowledge to medical research was made possible by the pioneer work of Sir Austin Bradford Hill. As a member of the scientific staff of the Medical Research Council he was the first to use central randomization in the multicentre trial of streptomycin in the treatment of pulmonary tuberculosis published in 1947.[2] His textbook, first written as a series of articles in the Lancet in the late 1930s, then published as 'Principles of Medical Statistics' and now (in its tenth edition) renamed 'A Short Text-book of Medical Statistics', remains a standard work.[3]

Selection of controls

Historical controls

When a new treatment has profoundly better results than the old treatment there is neither need nor ethical justification for a random control clinical trial; comparison with previous experience will suffice. The results of Semmelweis (mortality from puerperal sepsis in his unit fell from 11.4 per cent in 1846 to 1.3 per cent in 1848 after he introduced handwashing before examining patients in labour) and Lister (the use of the carbolic spray and dressings banished pyaemia, hospital gangrene and erysipelas from his wards) illustrate this, although pigheadedness and blind adherence to classical dogma prevented or delayed acceptance by their contemporaries. More recently, the treatment of bacterial endocarditis by penicillin and of leukaemia by cytotoxic drugs have been such great advances over previous experience that the use of other than historical controls would have been unethical.

Contemporary controls

Contemporary non-random controls

There are occasions when a new technique appears to be so much better than the one previously employed that it is allowable to compare its results with those of a matched group of contemporary patients, similar as far as possible except in that particular which is being tested. The widespread acceptance of monofilament non-absorbable sutures for closure of the aponeurosis after major laparotomies was a result of comparison with the high dehiscence rate after catgut closure, rather than of the results of random control trials.

Contemporary random controls

Many new treatments are, however, only marginally better than the old treatments; they may actually offer similar therapeutic results but be preferable from the points of view of cost, availability or ease of use. In such circumstances historical or contemporary non-random controls are not sufficient. The differences may be small, and the opportunities for bias large, and so the discipline of the random control trial is essential.[4, 5]

Proper conduct of random control trials (Fig. 10.1)

Planning a trial

If you are not honestly ignorant of the respective merits of the regimens concerned you must not enter a trial. The basis of the controlled trial is the null hypothesis – that there is no difference between the results of the two treatments under examination.

CLINICAL RESEARCH ALGORITHM

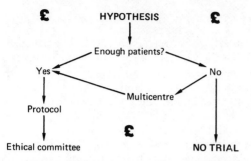

Fig. 10.1 Proper conduct of random control trials

Number of patients needed

If your trial is concerned with nominal data (success or failure), the calculation of how many patients you will need requires four numbers; first, you must cull from your records the rate of the event that you are proposing to study in those patients receiving your standard, or control, regimen. Secondly you must decide what percentage improvement would make you change your practice to the other, or 'experimental', regimen. The third and fourth numbers are predetermined figures, known as alpha and beta, which reduce the likelihood of the unjustified rejection, or unjustified acceptance, of the null hypothesis. Alpha is the probability of a false rejection of the null hypothesis and is usually set at less than 0.05, and beta is the probability of a false acceptance, set at either 0.10 or 0.20.

The following formula for the calculation is derived from Feinstein:[6]

$$\left(\frac{2.80}{P_1 - P_2}\right)^2 \left[P_1\,(100 - P_1) + P_2\,(100 - P_2)\right]$$

P_1 is the percentage of events in the control group. P_2 is the percentage of events in the experimental group which you would regard as sufficiently different to change your clinical practice. It allows alpha = 0.05 (a 5 per cent chance of falsely rejecting the null hypothesis) and beta = 0.20 (a 20 per cent chance of falsely accepting the null hypothesis). This is only an estimate, but so is the proportion you have decreed as clinically determinant, so a more accurate formula is not necessary.

The constant (which is the area in one [beta] plus two [alpha] tails of a standard normal curve) is as follows:

> 2.80 – alpha 0.05, beta 0.20
> 3.24 – alpha 0.05, beta 0.10
> 3.60 – alpha 0.02, beta 0.10
> 4.20 – alpha 0.01, beta 0.05

Example: The event rate in the control group is 20 per cent. A reduction to 10 per cent would be clinically determinant. Alpha = 0.05, beta = 0.20. The number in each arm of the trial should be:

$$\left(\frac{2.8}{20-10}\right)^2 \left[\, 20 \times (100-20) \,+\, 10 \times (100-10) \,\right] = 196$$

The assumption here is that alpha = 0.05 and beta = 0.20. It is also assumed that a clinically determinant outcome would be a halving of the event rate, although a reduction of one third may be acceptable. For other assumptions, other constants must be used.

If you conclude that you do not encounter sufficient patients to complete a trial within a reasonable time (2 years is the optimum), the choice is either to abandon the idea or organize a multi-centre trial.

Exclusions and withdrawals

More confusion possibly exists about the difference between exclusions and withdrawals than any other aspect of the organization of controlled trials. The distinction is, however, simple: exclusions are nominated before the start of a trial, are enumerated in the protocol, and these patients are not randomized. Withdrawals are those who are eligible for randomization but who, for whatever reason, do not achieve the end point specified. They may have been accidentally omitted from randomization, died before the specified time limit without an event having occurred, been lost to follow-up or for some other reason not followed protocol to the letter. Withdrawals must be recorded as zealously as the rest of the subjects in the trial, and analysed in the same way, though as a separate sub-group. Once a patient has been randomly allocated to a group, whatever happens to him he must be analysed as part of that group. It is only if the exclusions are specified, and the withdrawals analysed, that the results of a trial may be applied to the general population. Clinical trials, ideally, comprise a consecutive series of eligible patients.

Writing the protocol

The protocol should state the problem, your present practice, the theoretical justification for deviation from that practice, the safety of the proposed regimen, the group of patients you intend to study, the methods you are going to use and the manner in which you intend to inform patients and seek consent. It should also mention the way in which you intend to record, store, recall and analyse data.

This could form the 'Introduction' and 'Patients and Methods' sections of the paper. Now, of course, is the time to consult any medical or paramedical colleagues who may be involved and, if available, a biostatistician.

When the protocol has been approved by the Ethical Committee, a short summary of instructions should be written for those immediately involved in running the trial which lists their particular responsibilities.

Ethics

Bradford Hill's aphorism 'The ethical obligation always and entirely out-weighs the experimental' will have been at the forefront of your mind throughout the planning of the trial.[7] The control group will be guaranteed the best standard treatment; the experimental group will have the best standard treatment and differ only in the aspect you are testing. There is no place in clinical research for an 'untreated' control group. Placebos are only acceptable if they are prescribed in addition to the best standard treatment and as long as they do not harm the patient in any way; intramuscular injections of saline as placebos are indefensible.

No two clinicians will request informed consent in the same way, but the fundamental obligation is the same for all – that people should be fully informed of the potential risks and benefits of the proposed treatment and that their consent be freely obtained. No treatment will ever be given to a patient without his or her consent; the only issue is whether or not the fact of randomization should be disclosed. At present it seems to be generally accepted that if the regimen under trial is of no material concern to the patient (e.g. a trial of two antibiotics for wound infection prophylaxis, or two suture materials for wound closure) then the fact of randomization need not be disclosed but, if the regimen does materially affect the patient (e.g. lumpectomy or mastectomy for carcinoma) then the fact of randomization must be disclosed.

Design of the pro forma

The objectives of the trial should be considered at all times when designing the pro forma. Certain rules apply: the most important is – the simpler the form, the more likely it is to be completed. Secondly, it should fit in with the manner in which you are going to store, retrieve and analyse your data. If a computer will be involved, the form should be compatible. Once it is designed, you should test it in a pilot study and then print it on coloured paper so that it will be instantly recognizable.

Collecting and handling the data

Make sure that the forms are completed and checked without delay. Trying to answer missed questions months later is not rewarding. For a small trial, edge-punched cards with numerical codes may be adequate, but most people nowadays prefer to use a microcomputer. It takes a little longer to enter the data onto a floppy disk, but retrieval and analysis are infinitely quicker, particularly if you have a program which does exactly what is required.

It is important to monitor the progress of the trial personally. This will make sure that deviations from the protocol are kept to a minimum, that forms are properly filled in, and that the enthusiasm of co-workers is maintained and difficulties solved swiftly. A trial co-ordinator who checks pro formas, enters data, and keeps a system of filing which enables you to notice immediately if there have been any failures of randomization, or if any patient has failed to return for assessment or notes which have gone astray, is a great help.

Analysis of data

In this chapter I shall discuss only the analysis of nominal data. First one must divide the records into the groups being studied and compare the incidence of risk factors. The next step is to divide each group into 'event' and 'no event' and lay out a rough table.

From these figures it is possible to see whether or not there is a difference between the proportion of events in each group. It is necessary next to answer three questions. Could the difference have arisen by chance? What is the estimate of the true difference (the 95 per cent confidence limits)? Is the difference clinically important? The first two questions must be answered by statistical analysis, and I discuss the more common tests and the rules for their use in Chapter 11. The last question must be answered by common sense.

Once the appropriate test has been used to calculate the probability, it will be apparent whether the difference between the groups arose by chance. The conventional figure below which you can feel fairly confident that the difference did not arise by chance is 5 per cent ($P < 0.05$), but this is not an absolute; events which happen once in 20 times *do* happen once in 20 times, and you cannot assume that just because you have achieved what is known as 'statistical significance' you have found a true difference between your regimens.

Often the difference between the groups does not reach this level of significance. You then have to decide whether the difference is of clinical importance or not. If this level of significance has not been reached, the implication is that there are too few patients in the trial to justify acceptance of the null hypothesis. This can be demonstrated by calculation of the Type II (beta) error; the formula for this is the same as that used to calculate the numbers required for the trial. Even when the numbers have been calculated in advance, it is possible that the event rate in the control group may not tally with previous experience and so will invalidate that number.

Publishing the results of the trial

All reputable journals subscribe to the standard arrangement of *Introduction, Patients and Methods, Results, Discussion* and *Conclusion*, but each will have certain variations in layout and it is wise to consult the 'Instructions to Authors' of the journal to which you intend to submit your paper.

The *Introduction* must tell the reader why you did the trial. The *Patients and Methods* section must tell him – in sufficient detail for him to repeat the trial should he so wish – which group of patients you studied, definitions of end-points and your laboratory techniques. The *Results* section must convince him first that you have compared like with like and, secondly, that the difference or differences you report are really a result of the change in management you have tested. The *Discussion* should be succinct, and should put your work in the context of other work on that subject, and the *Conclusion* must be justified by the results you publish and not indulge in unsubstantiated conjecture.

Conclusion

Properly conducted random control clinical trials are valuable both for the assessment of new treatments and for the auditing of one's practice. They are costly in terms of time and money, both of which can be wasted by slovenly methods. These trials can, however, be not only useful but also immensely satisfying if done well.

References

1. Fisher RA. *Statistical Methods for Research Workers*. Edinburgh, Oliver and Boyd, 1925.
2. Medical Research Council. Streptomycin treatment of pulmonary tuberculosis. *Brit Med J* 1948; ii:769–82.
3. Bradford Hill A. *A Short Textbook of Medical Statistics*. London, Hodder and Stoughton, 1980.
4. Evans M, Pollock AV. A score system for evaluating random control clinical trials of prophylaxis of abdominal wound infection. *Brit J Surg* 1985; 72:256–60.
5. Pollock AV, Evans M. Bias and fraud in medical research: a review. *J Roy Soc Med* 1985; 78:937–40.
6. Feinstein AR. *Clinical Biostatistics*. St Louis, CV Mosby, 1977.
7. Bradford Hill A. Medical ethics and controlled trials. *Brit Med J* 1963; i:1043–49.

11

Statistics

Statistical significance of differences

Every random control clinical trial starts with a null hypothesis. The purpose of statistical analysis is to establish criteria for rejection or acceptance of that null hypothesis. It must be made perfectly clear that clinical relevance and statistical significance are two completely different things. If the numbers studied are large enough, it is easy to achieve statistical significance of a difference which in terms of the treatment of patients does not matter. If numbers are small, however, it may not be possible to attain statistical significance, although the difference is clinically important. The idea that a probability of less than 0.05 (there is less than one chance in 20 that the difference arose by chance) is 'significant' dates back to Ronald Fisher and is universally accepted. Healy, however, put this into perspective: 'It is a common misapprehension, reinforced by the use of the meaningless abbreviation 'NS' that the 5 per cent level of significance is some kind of absolute dividing line; it is, of course, wholly conventional'.[1]

A textbook of statistics cannot be condensed into one chapter, and you would be well-advised to buy, and keep in the office, two books; the first is Sir Austin Bradford Hill's 'A Short Textbook of Medical Statistics'.[2] This is the tenth edition of his famous 'Principles of Medical Statistics', which was first published in 1937. One of its (numerous) merits is that it is written in English, not in statistics. The second book is Sidney Siegel's 'Nonparametric Statistics for the Behavioral Sciences';[3] this is a mine of information on distribution-free statistical analysis. In the following sections I shall consider some of the simpler ways in which the statistical significance of differences can be assessed. Although I give the formulae for their calculation it is possible to do these tests on a programmable calculator or microcomputer.

Statistical analysis of proportions

The choice of tests

The analysis of pragmatic trials involves simple 'yes/no' answers. Did the patients in treatment group X suffer more events than those in group Y? There are two ways of calculating the statistical significance of these event/no event results. The tests are not interchangeable, and each one has its proper place. They are Fisher's exact probability test and the chi-square (χ^2) test. Both require the construction of a 2 × 2 contingency table, and the decision whether to use Fisher or χ^2 is made by considering the numbers in each treatment group.

The contingency table is constructed thus:

Event	Treatment group X A	Treatment group Y B	Total A + B
No-event	C	D	C + D
Total	A + C	B + D	A + B + C + D = N

The rule about the choice of tests is that if N is greater than 40 you may use the χ^2 test. If N is between 20 and 40 you may use the χ^2 test if the *expected* number in each cell is five or more, but if this figure is below five in any cell, you must use Fisher's test. If N is less than 20, you must always use Fisher's test. The formula for calculating the expected number is as follows:

$$\begin{array}{c|c} \dfrac{(A + C) \times (A + B)}{N} & \dfrac{(B + D) \times (A + B)}{N} \\ \hline \dfrac{(A + C) \times (C + D)}{N} & \dfrac{(B + D) \times (C + D)}{N} \end{array}$$

Take a hypothetical example. You have tested a new antibiotic against your previous standard for its ability to prevent wound infection in a trial comprising 38 colorectal operations. Eighteen patients have been given the new antibiotic, 20 have been given the standard antibiotic; there has been one wound infection in the 'new' group, and there have been eight wound infections in the 'old' group. The 2 × 2 contingency table looks like this:

	Treatment 'new'	Treatment 'old'	Total
Wound infection	1	8	9
No wound infection	17	12	29
Total	18	20	38

The expected numbers in each cell are:

$$\begin{array}{c|c} \dfrac{18 \times 9}{38} & \dfrac{20 \times 9}{38} \\ \hline \dfrac{18 \times 29}{38} & \dfrac{20 \times 29}{38} \end{array} = \begin{array}{c|c} 4.3 & 4.7 \\ \hline 13.7 & 15.3 \end{array}$$

Both cells A and B have expected numbers of less than five, therefore you must use Fisher's exact test, not the χ^2 test. The exact probability is 0.014.

Fisher's exact probability test

This gives the exact probability that the difference between two management regimens arose by chance. The formula involves factorials, for which the symbol is !; a factorial of a number is that number multiplied by the next lower number, multiplied by the next lower number, and so on. For example, the factorial of 4 (4!) is 4 × 3 × 2 × 1 = 24. The factorial of 0 is accepted as 1 (as is that of 1). The arithmetic can involve very large numbers unless a short cut which is mentioned below is adopted. The formula for Fisher's exact test is:

$$P = \frac{(A + B)! \ (C + D)! \ (A + C)! \ (B + D)!}{N! \ A! \ B! \ C! \ D!}$$

(A, B, C, D are the cells, and N is the total in the 2 × 2 contingency table).

The following example is taken from James Lind's 'Treatise of the Scurvy' published in 1753.[4] In 1747 'on board the Salisbury at sea' he treated 12 patients with scurvy. 'Their cases were as similar as I could have them'. Two who were given oranges and lemons were cured, the others were not. The contingency table is:

	Oranges and lemons	Other treatment	Total
Cured	(A) 2	(B) 0	(A + B) 2
Not cured	(C) 0	(D) 10	(C + D) 10
Total	(A + C) 2	(B + D) 10	N 12

$$\text{Fisher's test } P = \frac{2! \ 10! \ 2! \ 10!}{12! \ 2! \ 0! \ 0! \ 10!}$$

If this is calculated directly:

$$P = \frac{2 \times 3628800 \times 2 \times 3628800}{479001600 \times 2 \times 1 \times 1 \times 3628800}$$

There are too many figures here for the average calculator, but the sum can easily be calculated by cancelling equal numbers in the numerator and denominator:

$$P = \frac{2 \times 1 \times 10 \times 9 \times 8 \times 7 \times 6 \times 5 \times 4 \times 3 \times 2 \times 1 \times 2 \times 1 \times 10 \times 9 \times 8 \times 7 \times 6 \times 5 \times 4 \times 3 \times 2 \times 1}{12 \times 11 \times 10 \times 9 \times 8 \times 7 \times 6 \times 5 \times 4 \times 3 \times 2 \times 1 \times 2 \times 1 \times 1 \times 1 \times 10 \times 9 \times 8 \times 7 \times 6 \times 5 \times 4 \times 3 \times 2 \times 1}$$

By cancellation this becomes:

$$P = \frac{2}{12 \times 11} = \frac{2}{132} = 0.015$$

Often the number of figures in a Fisher equation defeats the capacity of a calculator, even after cancellation. In this case, a sensible trick is to cut up the formula and not to try to enter the full numerator and divide it by the full denominator. Here is an example from a recent publication.[5] Two patients out of 17 in one arm of the trial suffered a surgical wound infection compared with 8 out of 21 in the other. The contingency table reads:

	Group I	Group II	Total
Wound infection	2	8	10
No wound infection	15	13	28
Total	17	21	38

The χ^2 test is inappropriate as the expected number in one cell is less than five:

$$\frac{17 \times 10}{38} = 4.47$$

Fisher's test gives the following equation:

$$P = \frac{10! \ 28! \ 17! \ 21!}{38! \ 2! \ 8! \ 15! \ 13!}$$

By cancellation this becomes:

$$P = \frac{10 \times 9 \times 17 \times 16 \times 21 \times 20 \times 19 \times 18 \times 17 \times 16 \times 15 \times 14}{38 \times 37 \times 36 \times 35 \times 34 \times 33 \times 32 \times 31 \times 30 \times 29 \times 2}$$

It can easily be calculated with a pocket calculator as follows:

$$P = 10 \div 38 \times 9 \div 37 \times 17 \div 36 \times 16 \div 35 \times 21 \div 34 \times 20 \div 33 \times 19$$
$$\div 32 \times 18 \div 31 \times 17 \div 30 \times 16 \div 29 \times 15 \div 2 \times 14$$
$$P = 0.0585$$

It is usual to make a correction to the Fisher test when the value in one of the cells is greater than zero. In this case further contingency tables are prepared with more extreme results and the test is repeated. The true (corrected) probability is the sum of all the probabilities calculated. In the trial quoted above, the correction factors are calculated after rewriting the contingency tables thus:

	Group I	Group II	Total
Wound infection	1	9	10
No wound infection	16	12	28
Total	17	21	38

and

	Group I	Group II	Total
Wound infection	0	10	10
No wound infection	17	11	28
Total	17	21	38

The correcting equations are as follows:

$$P = \frac{10! \ 28! \ 17! \ 21!}{38! \ 1! \ 9! \ 16! \ 12!}$$
$$P = 0.0106$$

and

$$P = \frac{10! \ 28! \ 17! \ 21!}{38! \ 0! \ 10! \ 17! \ 11!}$$
$$P = 0.0007$$
$$\text{Corrected } P = 0.0585 + 0.0106 + 0.0007$$
$$= 0.0698$$

Chi-square test

It is usual when using this test in comparing the results of two regimens to incorporate Yates's correction for continuity. The correction is applied not, as some people believe, for small numbers of patients. It is the small number of groups (two) being compared which some statisticians regard as an indication for its use. The following formula incorporates Yates's correction $(-\frac{N}{2})$. The sign $|\quad|$ means the difference between two values; the smaller number is always substracted from the larger.

$$\chi^2 = \frac{N(|AD - BC| - \frac{N}{2})^2}{(A + B)(C + D)(A + C)(B + D)}$$

The symbols used are those of the 2 × 2 contingency table).
Having worked out the value of χ^2, P is determined by looking up the tables for one degree of freedom. The important figures are 3.84 (above which $P <$ 0.05), 5.41 ($P < 0.02$), 6.63 ($P < 0.01$) and 10.83 ($P < 0.001$).

Confidence limits or intervals

As an addition to the χ^2 or Fisher test of the significance of differences, it is valuable to calculate the limits within which a difference in the outcome of two regimens can be regarded, with 95 per cent confidence, as lying. Wide confidence intervals suggest that the sample is too small, and warn against too ready an acceptance of the results, whether 'statistically significant', or not. The formula is:

$$|P_1 - P_2| \pm 1.96 \sqrt{\left(\frac{P_1 Q_1}{N_1} + \frac{P_2 Q_2}{N_2}\right)}$$

P_1 = the proportion of patients in whom an event occurs in one management group.
P_2 = the proportion of patients in whom an event occurs in the other management group.
Q_1 = the proportion of patients in whom the event does not occur in one management group.
Q_2 = the proportion of patients in whom the event does not occur in the other management group.
N_1 = the number of patients in the first group.
N_2 = the number of patients in the second group.
We will use the same results which we used to exemplify Fisher's test.[4] The figures are:

$$P_1 = 0.118: P_2 = 0.381: Q_1 = 0.882: Q_2 = 0.619: N_1 = 17: N_2 = 21$$

The confidence limits are:

$$0.263 \pm 1.96 \sqrt{0.0061 + 0.0112} = 0.263 \pm 1.96 \times 0.1315$$
$$= 0.263 \pm 0.258$$
$$= 0.005 \text{ to } 0.521$$

The 95 per cent confidence limits are, therefore, 0.5 per cent to 52.1 per cent in favour of Group I. This means that the results must be accepted with caution (just as the exact *P* value of 0.0698 must be). If the confidence limits include a negative proportion, the results cannot be accepted as statistically significant.

Confidence intervals are equally valuable when considering the differences between means. The 95 per cent confidence intervals of a mean are approximately between two standard errors above and two standard errors below that mean.

Statistical analysis of numbers

Usually, in addition to answering the principal question posed by the trial, data of an explanatory nature need to be analyzed and published. For example, did the patients in one treatment group stay longer in hospital? Was the duration of postoperative pyrexia longer?

Analysis by Student's 't' test

The overriding rule for the use of this simple and strong test is that your data must have a 'normal' or Gaussian distribution. To calculate the '*t*' test you will have to determine certain values. These are the mean (often written $\bar{x}$, pronounced x-bar), the standard deviation (often written δ, pronounced sigma), the standard error of the mean (often written s.e.m.) and the median.

The **mean** of a series of values is the sum of all those values divided by the number of observations.

The **standard deviation** is the square root of the variance. The formula is:

$$\sqrt{\left(\frac{\text{sum of x}^2 - \dfrac{(\text{sum of x})^2}{n}}{n-1} \right)}$$

X is the numerical value of each observation and N is the number of observations.

The **standard error of the mean** is the standard deviation divided by the square root of the number of observations.

$$\text{s.e.m.} = \frac{\delta}{\sqrt{n}}$$

The **median** is the value above and below which an equal number of observations lie.

If data are not normally distributed, they are called 'skewed', and there are several ways of determining skewness. First, you may plot the values you have found in your trial against the number of patients (many microcomputers will do this). If the resulting curve is obviously not bell-shaped, you will be well-advised to eschew the '*t*' test and opt for one of the nonparametric tests. Secondly, if the value of the mean differs considerably from that of the median, you can be sure you are not dealing with a normal distribution. Thirdly, if the standard deviation is more than half the value of the mean, the distribution is skewed.

Most biological data are not normally distributed. Hall studied 72 papers published in the *British Journal of Surgery* in 1979 and 1980 which used a 't' test for statistical analysis.[6] He found that two thirds of them made unjustified assumptions about normality and should not have been analysed by the 't' test.

Calculation of the Student's 't' test

The formula is:

$$t = \frac{\text{difference between the means}}{\text{standard error of the difference}}$$

The standard error of the difference is:

$$\sqrt{(\text{s.e.m. of Group I})^2 + (\text{s.e.m. of Group II})^2}$$

As a rule of thumb, in trials comprising more than 30 patients, if the difference between the means exceeds twice the standard error of the difference, then it is statistically significant. Tables for the conversion of '*t*' to probability are given in most textbooks of statistics.

Non-parametric tests of the significance of differences between groups

There are two ways of dealing with numbers which are not normally distributed. First, they may be transformed logarithmically, which can achieve normality. This is the device used by the Statistical Package for the Social Sciences (SPSS) which is designed for mainframe computer analysis, and allows the 'strong' parametric tests to be used. The second method is to rank the numbers and then use one of the newer, but somewhat weaker, non-parametric tests. Non-parametric tests are discussed in detail in Siegel's book;[3] I will confine myself to discussion of three methods of solving the problem which is most frequently encountered – the statistical comparison of two independent samples.

Analysis by chi-square test

Set an arbitrary line and then analyze the data by the χ^2 test for 2×2 contingencies. Thus you may divide hospital stay into two categories, 0–9 days, and 10 days or more. It is a crude method and may fail to uncover clinically important differences between treatment groups. It is often useful, however, in discovering risk factors. For example, you may have observed that young obese patients suffer more wound infections after contaminated operations than young thin patients. In investigating the validity of this observation one must define obesity as, for example, a thickness of subcutaneous abdominal wall fat of 2.5 cm or more, measured during the operation at the site of incision, and define 'young' as under the age of

65 years. This allows you to draw up a simple 2 × 2 contingency table and use the χ^2 test for analysis.

We found the following results in patients whose subcutaneous tissues had been contaminated by intestinal bacteria during operation:[7]

Wound infection	Young obese 30	Young thin 19
No wound infection	45	110

$$\chi^2 = 16.69, P < 0.001$$

The median test

This is another simple method of analysis. It involves arranging in a 2 × 2 contingency table the number of values in each group lying above the median of the two groups amalgamated, and the number of values at or below the combined median, and then analysing the result by either a chi-square or Fisher's exact test. Most valid controlled trials will involve at least 100 patients but, for the sake of simplicity I will give the following hypothetical example of the duration of postoperative stay after two methods of management in just 15 patients. The number of days in management group X were: 3, 3, 4, 4, 4, 6 and 8; in group Y they were 4, 5, 9, 14, 20, 23, 35 and 36. The combined median is 6 and the contingency table looks like this:

	Group X	Group Y	Total
Above median	1	6	7
At or below median	6	2	8
Total	7	8	15

Fisher's test:

$$P = \frac{7! \times 8! \times 7! \times 8!}{15! \times 1! \times 6! \times 6! \times 2!}$$
$$= 0.03$$

The Mann–Whitney 'U' test

This was introduced in 1947 and is widely used in analysing numerical data in biological research. The essential steps are as follows:

1. Rank the numbers in both arms of the trial together from one to N (the total number of patients in the trial). Equal numbers are given the average rank, so that the highest rank equals the total number of patients.
2. Sum the ranks in each arm separately.
3. Call the number of observations in the arm with the smaller sum of ranks n_1, the number of observations in the other arm n_2, and the respective sums of ranks R_1 and R_2.
4. Calculate 'U' from the formula:

$$U = n_1 n_2 + \frac{n_1 (n_1 + 1)}{2} - R_1$$

5. Calculate z from the formula:

$$z = \frac{U - \dfrac{n_1 n_2}{2}}{\sqrt{\left\{ \dfrac{n_1 n_2 (n_1 + n_2 + 1)}{12} \right\}}}$$

6. Look up the tables (Siegel, 1956, page 247)[3] the probability of z being as large as it is by chance. The important figures are: $z = 1.65, P < 0.05$: $z = 2.06, P < 0.02$: $z = 2.33, P < 0.01$ and $z = 3.11$, $P < 0.001$.

An example of the Mann-Whitney 'U' test follows. Forty patients were randomly allocated to one of two management regimens. Their postoperative stay in hospital ranged between 3 and 46 days, and the numbers of days were ranked as shown below.

Management regimen X		Management regimen Y	
Number of days	Rank	Number of days	Rank
3	2	4	6
3	2	6	14
3	2	6	14
4	6	6	14
4	6	8	22
4	6	8	22
4	6	8	22
5	9.5	8	22
5	9.5	9	25.5
6	14	9	25.5
6	14	10	27
6	14	11	28.5
6	14	15	30
7	18.5	18	31
7	18.5	25	33
8	22	26	34
11	28.5	27	35
22	32	29	36
$n_1 = 18$	$R_1 = 222.5$	32	37
		35	38
		39	39
		46	40
		$n_2 = 22$	$R_2 = 595.5$

$$U = 18 \times 22 + \frac{18 \times 19}{2} - 222.5$$
$$= 344.5$$
$$z = \frac{344.5 - 198}{\sqrt{1353}}$$
$$= 3.98 \qquad P < 0.0001$$

Tests of correlation

In the context of controlled clinical trials tests of the relationship between two sets of measurement are seldom useful, but if you are going to use correlation tests you must be absolutely certain that the two sets are indepen- dent of each other. Thus, it is of little value to produce a correlation coefficient of measurements of urea content against creatinine content in the blood, as they both measure renal function. Most of the correlations which you can demonstrate in the course of your controlled trial (e.g. that fat people suffer more wound infections than thin people) are best stated without recourse to correlation calculations.

Biological behaviour is conditioned by so many factors that simple corre- lation is seldom justified, and multiple regression calculations are fashion- able. They are, however, disappointing in that the equation derived from one set of observations can seldom be generalized for the whole population.

If you think that two independent measurements are correlated, it is best to start by constructing a scattergram. The closer the correlation the nearer the dots will be to making a straight line, and the more likely it is that your two sets of observations are correlated. You may then calculate the coeffi- cient of correlation (r) by adding all the deviations from the mean in one set of observations, multiplying by the sum of all the deviations in the other set, and dividing the answer by the product of the standard deviations in each set. Thus:

$$r = \frac{\text{sum }(x - \bar{x})\,\text{sum }(y - \bar{y})}{\delta x \,\delta y}$$

The more nearly r approaches $+1$ or -1, the closer the correlation between the two sets of observations will be. The correlation may, of course, be positive (the greater the value of x, the greater the value of y) or negative (the greater the value of x, the less the value of y). The probability that a correla- tion has arisen by chance can be calculated by deriving a 't' value from the formula (numerator and denominator as in the formula for r given above):

$$t = \sqrt{\left\{\frac{(n-2)\,\text{numerator}^2}{\text{denominator}^2 - \text{numerator}^2}\right\}}$$

P is given in the tables of 't'.

The Type II error

The Type I error, known as alpha, is the unjustified **rejection** of the null hypothesis. Most of the statistical tests which we have considered so far are directed towards minimizing this error.

The Type II, or beta, error is the unjustified **acceptance** of the null hypothesis. Many controlled clinical trials are published which show no statistically significant differences between the groups. What we are inter- ested in is the question – is there a clinically important difference between them and, if so, how many more patients would be needed to show whether or not this difference arose by chance?

Whereas we accept $P < 0.05$ (alpha $= 0.05$, a 95 per cent probability) in rejecting the null hypothesis, it is customary to accept beta $= 0.20$, or 0.10

(80 per cent or 90 per cent chance) that our results do mean that there is no difference between the two arms of the trial, and that the null hypothesis can be accepted. The formula which follows is the one we used in calculating the number of patients required in a clinical trial. It is derived from tables of the normal deviate and specifies a 5 per cent chance of a false positive result (Type I error) and a 10 per cent chance of a false negative result (Type II error).

$$n = \left(\frac{1.96 + 1.28}{P_1 - P_2}\right)^2 \{P_1(100 - P_1) + P_2(100 - P_2)\}$$

n = the number of patients required in each arm of the trial
P_1 = the percentage of events in Group 1
P_2 = the percentage of events in Group 2

Published reports of controlled clinical trials which show no statistically significant difference in the percentage of events between the two groups rarely mention the Type II error. I give an example selected at random from recent publications on antibiotic prophylaxis of abdominal surgical wound infection. The authors randomized 77 patients into two groups.[8] Patients in Group 1 were given a single dose of 600 mg doxycycline pre-operatively, patients in Group 2 were given the same dose postoperatively. They reported 3 wound infections out of 42 in Group 1 (7.1 per cent) and 7 out of 35 in Group 2 (20.0 per cent). Fisher's test gives an exact probability of 0.0638, and the null hypothesis cannot be rejected with confidence. On the basis of these percentages (the difference between which is clearly important), however, the null hypothesis cannot be accepted. In order to satisfy alpha = 0.05 and beta = 0.10, each arm of the trial should have had n patients:

$$n = \left(\frac{3.24}{12.9}\right)^2 \{(7.1 \times 92.9) + (20 \times 80)\}$$
$$= 0.06308 \times 2260 = 142.6$$

If, on the other hand, the difference in the percentage of events in each arm is so small that it is of no clinical importance, there is no point in extending the trial until statistical significance is achieved.

References

1. Healy MJR. Yes, no and maybe. *Br Med J* 1983; **286**:1445.
2. Bradford Hill A. *A Short Textbook of Medical Statistics*. London, Hodder and Stoughton Educational, 1977.
3. Siegel S. *Nonparametric Statistics for the Behavioral Sciences*. Tokyo, McGraw Hill Kogakusha, 1956.
4. Lind J. *A Treatise of the Scurvy*. Edinburgh, Kincaid and Donaldson, 1753.
5. Hagen TB, Bergan T, Liavåg I. Prophylactic metronidazole in elective colorectal surgery. *Acta Chir Scand* 1980; **146**:71–5.
6. Hall JC. Use of the "t" test in the British Journal of Surgery. *Br J Surg* 1982; **69**:55–56.
7. Pollock AV, Evans M. Postoperative wound infection: the influence of age and obesity. *SE Asia J Surg* 1984; **7**:243–47.
8. Törnqvist A, Ekelund G, Forsgren A, Leandoer L, Olson S, Ursing J. Single-dose doxycycline prophylaxis and peroperative bacteriological culture in elective colorectal surgery. *Br J Surg* 1981; **68**:565–68.

Part IV

Community-acquired Surgical Infections

12

Burns

'The control of infection in burns involves a battle of human wits against microbial genes'.[1] A burn, by its very nature, is sterile, and if it gets infected, the causative organisms are acquired in the hospital and not in the community. The outcome of a burn depends on both the **extent** and the **depth** of the wound. The main cause of death in fires is, however, not the burn, but the inhalation of carbon monoxide and smoke, particularly if the fire involves certain plastic fibres which give off highly toxic fumes when they burn. The percentage of body surface burned can be judged with reasonable accuracy by applying the 'rule of nine' (Fig. 12.1) Roughly, the front and back of the torso and the whole of each lower limb are all 18 per cent, the head and each upper limb are all 9 per cent. These percentages vary with age, the head being relatively much bigger in infants.

It is important to distinguish between partial and full-thickness skin loss. The former will heal by re-epithelialization from intact dermal cells either of the deeper layers of the skin or of the hair follicles and sweat or sebaceous glands. Full-thickness skin loss, however, in the absence of surgical treatment, can only heal by the slow ingrowth of epithelial cells from the edges of the burn.

Although the judgement of the extent of a burn is easy, that of its depth is often difficult in the first few days. All electrical burns, most flame burns, most freeze burns (and many scalds in children) are full-thickness. Infection in a partial-skin-loss burn converts it into a full-thickness burn. The judgement of the extent is made mainly by inspection: erythema and blistering signify partial destruction, whereas a full-thickness burn soon becomes discoloured and insensitive to pin-prick. Disulphine blue (10 ml) injected intravenously stains normal skin and partial thickness, but not full-thickness, burns.

Metabolic effects of burns

Fluid, electrolyte and protein loss

Capillaries in the subcutaneous tissue under a burn are damaged and rendered permeable to fluid, electrolytes and plasma proteins, resulting in hypovolaemic shock; the more extensive the burn, the greater the shock. Records of the Glasgow Royal Infirmary during 1937–1941 showed that 72 per cent of burn deaths occurred within 3 days.[2] This outcome was radically changed by the introduction of intravenous fluid infusions for any burn involving more than 10 per cent of body surface in children and 20 per cent in adults.

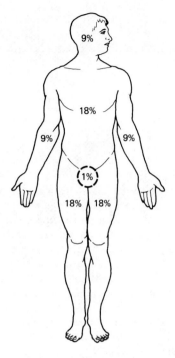

Fig. 12.1 Wallace's rule of 9

Whether the fluid should contain electrolytes alone (Ringer lactate) or whether colloids such as dextran or plasma should be added is still controversial. As Shoemaker and Hauser wrote 'These questions are not answered by simplistic notions based on anecdotal incidents of extreme cases, party-line philosophical theories, or inadequately controlled series by protagonists of a particular point of view'.[3]

Whatever fluid you use for replacement, the estimation of the volume required is not easy. Severely burned patients can sequester enormous quantities in the subcutaneous tissues, and the best guide to the adequacy of fluid replacement is not urine output, which may reflect pituitary antidiuretic secretion rather than volume deficit, but stability of the circulation. Formulae such as twice the weight in kilograms (e.g. 140 ml for a 70 kg patient) for each per cent of the burn in the first 8 hours, and a similar quantity in the next 16 hours, are useful as rough guides.[4]

Effects of burns on host defence mechanisms

The ability of the burned patient to resist microbial invasion is reduced in many ways.

Tissue anoxia

Both systemic and local factors can interfere with tissue oxygenation in severe burns. On the one hand, carbon monoxide inhalation, hypovolaemia and lung damage from smoke inhalation and, on the other hand, local vascular occlusion, play their part in causing tissue anoxia which is possibly the most important cause of the reduction in immune competence of severely burned patients. Correction of hypovolaemia and arterial anoxia are essential. Oxygen should be administered by mask or, in extreme cases, by endotracheal intubation and positive pressure ventilation. Both volume repletion and arterial oxygenation must be monitored, the former by central venous or Swan-Gantz catheter and the latter by frequent arterial blood gas analyses. If rapid infusion of 1 litre of saline does not considerably raise the central venous or pulmonary capillary wedge pressure, that litre and more are needed.

Defects in cellular and humoral defences

The defence capabilities of neutrophils, lymphocytes and monocytes are all depressed in patients with severe burns, not only because of loss of normal components of the defence system, but also as a result of the action of toxic products. Chemotaxis, phagocytosis and intracellular killing of bacteria are defective, the serum levels of immunoglobulins and complement fall, and the ability of T-lymphocytes to stimulate production of antibodies by B-lymphocytes is reduced. The anergy of severely burned patients is shown by absence of skin reactivity to recall antigens and by the patient's acceptance, for up to 3 weeks, of allografts of skin. All injuries are followed by negative nitrogen balance; protein catabolism is a feature of severe burns, and it is aggravated by infection.

Prevention of infection in burned patients

This depends on three things: prevention of microbial colonization, prevention of microbial invasion and assistance of host defences. The organisms most frequently isolated from burn wounds are *Staphylococcus aureus, Pseudomonas aeruginosa* and coliforms.[5] *Streptococcus pyogenes* is rare, but it is of special importance because it will kill skin grafts. *Clostridium tetani* is even rarer, but it is so important that all patients with deep burns should be given a single dose of one mega-unit of penicillin intramuscularly when they are first seen.

Prevention of microbial colonization

A burn is a sterile wound, and it would heal without infection if we could prevent bacteria (and, rarely, other microorganisms) coming into contact with it. Microbial colonization is, however, common in all full-thickness burns. Most of these nosocomial infections are of exogenous origin, and burned patients should be nursed in single-bed rooms with plenum ventilation by outside or filtered air.[6] Airborne contamination is, however, less important than that which is introduced on the hands of attendants, and strict handwashing rituals should be practised.

A small burn can be protected by applying an adhesive polyurethane membrane which is permeable to gases but not to bacteria. The idea of totally isolating the burned patient in a clean air enclosure is attractive, it but does not overcome the problem of colonization by organisms from the patient's own skin or gut.[7, 8]

Prevention of microbial invasion

Creating an antimicrobial barrier

As our best efforts cannot entirely keep a burn wound from becoming colonized, we must seek methods to prevent bacteria from invading the tissues. We do this by forming an antimicrobial barrier over the surface of the burn. In the 1930s this was achieved by the application of tannic acid which formed an impervious eschar. It was, however, partly absorbed, and was thought to cause liver necrosis. Since its abandonment, many alternatives have been tried, all of which create more or less efficient barriers. In certain circumstances such as moderate-sized burns on less than half the circumference of limb or trunk, the exposure treatment introduced by Wallace in 1951 is effective; it allows the formation of an impervious scab under which healing can proceed.[9]

Many antibiotics have been applied to the surface of burns, but problems have always arisen as a result of emergence of strains of bacteria which are resistant to the antibiotics used. This phenomenon is less likely to occur with the use of modern chemical barriers; mafenide acetate cream is effective, but can exacerbate acidosis. Silver nitrate is expensive in terms of spoiled linen, and the preferred topical agent nowadays is silver-sulphadiazine cream applied daily and covered by sterile dressings and bandages.

The role of excision and grafting

Surgeons who favour tangential excision and grafting between the third and fifth days after a burn, recognize the undoubted superiority of skin as an antimicrobial barrier,[10] which is particularly applicable to burns of the hands and eyelids. On the other hand, it is difficult to be sure so soon after a burn that it *is* full-thickness and, secondly, extensive excisions and the taking of split skin grafts can cause a lot of bleeding at a stage when the patient's haemodynamic state may still be unstable. When the burn is so extensive that it is impossible to take enough grafts from unburned skin, the use of meshed autografts can double the area covered. Cadaver allografts may survive for as long as 3 weeks, and give time for the growth of cultures from fragments of the patient's own skin.[11] This exciting development, pioneered by Howard Green in Boston, USA, offers the possibility of rescuing patients with even near-total skin destruction. The cultured skin is, however, fragile and easily digested by bacteria. The tissue on which it is placed must be as nearly sterile as possible. Achauer and his colleagues published a case report of an 11-year-old boy with 85 per cent fire burns who was allografted with frozen banked skin and treated with cyclosporin 8 mg/Kg/day for 4 months.[12] Two years later the allografts were complete and there was no sign of rejection.

Assisting host defences

There are certain obvious defects which we must correct. We can ensure that tissue oxygenation is maintained, we can give blood transfusions for anaemia, and we must prescribe antacids or H_2 antagonists to protect the stomach against stress ulcers.

Extensive burns deplete reserves of body protein in two ways. First, the exudate from the burned surface is plasma, and large quantities of plasma proteins are lost in that way. Secondly, there is a prolonged catabolic phase following burns. In the absence of sepsis this may continue for 3 or 4 weeks and result in the loss of 10 per cent of body weight. In the presence of sepsis the process accelerates and weight losses up to 30 per cent are encountered.

It is not feasible to supply the amount of calories and protein which the body requires by increasing oral intake, which merely results in vomiting and diarrhoea. There is, however, a clinical impression that aggressive feeding results in a smoother recovery. Work in J. Wesley Alexander's department[13] supports this view and encourages us to use fine-tube nasogastric infusion of high-calorie high-protein fluids. The place of intravenous hyperalimentation is less well-defined, and sepsis associated with central venous catheters is more of a problem in burns than in other conditions such as high intestinal fistulas for which it is used.

We know of no way of stimulating phagocytosis, fibroblast proliferation or epithelial growth. We cannot at present, persuade B-lymphocytes to form more antibodies. Polyvalent anti-pseudomonas vaccines and sera have bene-fited burned children in New Delhi,[14] and there is hope that a common bacterial surface antigen such as J5 may prove useful in assisting the body's humoral defences against infection.[15]

Detection and treatment of burn wound sepsis

As the body's defence mechanisms are defective when a large area of skin is destroyed, the classical signs of inflammation are usually absent and other signs of microbial invasion must be sought. Clinical experience is an ade-quate guide: a patient who, after apparently doing well, refuses food and becomes somewhat irrational is probably suffering from sepsis and requires urgent antibiotic treatment. An important local indicator is the conversion of partial thickness to full-thickness skin destruction. Repeated blood cul-tures are valuable, but culture of the surface of the burn reveals the nature of colonists, not necessarily of invaders. For this reason Pruitt recommends frequent biopsies under local anaesthesia with immediate Gram-staining and quantitative culture.[16] One or more bacterium per high-power field in living tissue or 10^5 or more per gram of tissue indicates infection. In the presence of infection, Pruitt advises the subeschar injection, with a spinal needle, of an appropriate antibiotic prior to excision and grafting. It is for the treatment of established infection, and only for the treatment of established infection, that systemic antibiotics are required. Prophylactic antibiotics (except for a single dose of penicillin for the prevention of tetanus) can do nothing more than encourage the invasion of resistant strains.

Conclusions

The principles of burn treatment are:

1. the correction of hypovolaemia and tissue anoxia,
2. the recognition that bacterial colonization derives mainly from attendants' hands,
3. the provision of an antimicrobial barrier on the wound,
4. the early detection and treatment of invasive infection,
5. the early covering of the wound with autologous skin,
6. nutritional support, either enterally or parenterally.

Topical antibiotics should never be used, and systemic antibiotics only for the treatment of an infection, the causative organism of which has been defined.

References

1. Lowbury EJL. Wits versus genes. The continuing battle against infection. *J Trauma* 1977; **19**:33–45.
2. Jackson D McG. Burns: McIndoe's contribution and subsequent advances. *Ann Roy Coll Surg Eng* 1979; **61**:335–340.
3. Shoemaker WC and Hauser CJ. Critique of crystalloid versus colloid therapy in shock and shock lung. *Crit Care Med* 1979; **7**:117–124.
4. Baxter CR. Fluid volume and electrolyte changes in the early post burn period. *Clin Plast Surg* 1974; **1**:693–96.
5. Laurence JC. The bacteriology of burns. *J Hosp Infect* 1985; **6**(suppl B):3–17.
6. Bourdillon RB and Colebrook L. Air hygeine in dressing-rooms for burns or major wounds. *Lancet* 1946; **i**:561–565 and 601–605.
7. Minns RJ and Carter R. A portable clean air enclosure for neutropenic patients requiring hospital treatment: a preliminary study. *J Hosp Infect* 1983; **4**:406–409.
8. Scott JM, McLaughlan J and Smylie HG. Sterile microenvironment in prevention of wound infection. *Brit Med J* 1982; **284**:1594–1596.
9. Wallace AB. The exposure treatment of burns. *Lancet* 1951; **i**:501–504.
10. Tolhurst DE. The treatment of burns. *Ann Roy Coll Surg Engl* 1980; **62**:120–124.
11. Gallico CG, O'Connor NE, Compton CC, Kehinde O, Green H. Permanent coverage of large burn wounds with autologous human epithelium. *New Eng J Med* 1984; **311**:448–451.
12. Achauer BM, Hewitt CW, Blacks KS *et al.* Long-term skin allograft survival after short-term cyclosporin treatment in a patient with massive burns. *Lancet* 1986; **1**:14–15.
13. Alexander JW, MacMillan BG, Spinnett SD *et al.* Beneficial effects of aggressive protein feeding in severely burned children. *Ann Surg* 1980; **192**:505–507.
14. Jones RJ, Roe EA and Gupta JL. Controlled trial of pseudomonas immunoglobulin and vaccine in burn patients. *Lancet* 1980; **ii**:1263–1265.
15. Baumgartner J-D, Glauser MP, McCutchan JA *et al.* Prevention of Gram-negative shock and death in surgical patients by antibody to endotoxin core glycolipid. *Lancet* 1985; **ii**:59–63.
16. Pruitt BA. Biopsy diagnosis of surgical infections. *New Eng J Med* 1984; **310**:1737–1738.

13

Infections following blunt trauma

The damage to the body done by a blow is proportional to the square of the velocity of impact: kinetic energy = mass × square of velocity. It is therefore obvious that the greater the speed of a motor vehicle or the height of a fall, the more likelihood there is of skin or mucous membrane splitting and so allowing harmless resident bacteria to invade the tissues.

In dealing with these injuries the principles are few but compelling: it is essential that the hypovolaemia is corrected, an antibiotic is administered immediately, the break in the integument is repaired speedily, and every effort is made to avoid additional exogenous bacterial contamination.

Lacerations as a result of blunt trauma

Wherever the skin is separated from the underlying bone by less than 5–10 mm of subcutaneous tissue there is a strong chance that a blow will split the skin and cause a laceration. As a rule these lacerations can be treated by debridement and suture, but there is a special case – the elderly person who receives a blow on the shin resulting in an L-shaped wound. The blood supply to the flap is so poor that it usually dies, allowing the development of secondary infection. It is far better in these cases to excise most of the flap and cover the defect with a split skin graft when the patient is first seen. This can save weeks of dressings and avoid the possibility of graft failure on an infected bed.

Compound fractures

As soon as possible after the accident the patient should be given an effective antibiotic parenterally. The bacteria which may contaminate such a fracture are derived not only from the patient's skin but also, potentially, from exogenous sources – clothing, road dirt or the hands of attendants. A suitable antibiotic, would therefore, be a second-generation cephalosporin, such as cefazolin, which can control both Gram-positive and Gram-negative organisms.[1] At the same time the skin wound should be protected from futher contamination by the application of sterile dressings, and the patient should be given a booster dose of tetanus toxoid.

Operation must be undertaken as soon as hypovolaemia has been corrected. Foreign bodies, and devitalized tissues, must be excised and the fracture reduced and immobilized, which may require internal fixation by screws, plates or nails. The skin can usually be closed unless there has been extensive skin loss or devitalization, or gross delay before operation. No more than two further doses of antibiotic should be given; there is no theoretical or experimental support for the practice of continuing prophylactic antibiotics beyond 24 hours.

Intestinal perforation as a result of blunt abdominal trauma

Any part of the intestine may be ruptured by a blow; the relatively fixed parts, the duodenum, duodeno-jejunal flexure and ileo-caecal region are most at risk. Furthermore, the mesentery or mesocolon may be torn off the intestine, resulting in gangrene and perforation. The compulsory wearing of seat belts in Britain and other countries has saved many lives which would otherwise have been wasted as a result of head injuries, but the seat belt itself can cause intestinal rupture. The early diagnosis of such an injury is never easy, particularly in a patient who also has a head or chest injury. The prognosis after early laparotomy is, however, so much better than if laparotomy is delayed that every effort must be made to diagnose significant damage to the intestine or to other intra-abdominal organs. In these patients I find that a 1 litre saline peritoneal lavage is very useful. If the returning peritoneal fluid is blood-stained, and particularly if the ratio of leucocytes to red cells in the stained sediment after lavage is more than 1:10, immediate laparotomy is indicated.[2]

The patient should be given 500 mg of metronidazole together with either 1 g of a cephalosporin or 120 mg gentamicin intravenously as soon as the decision for laparotomy has been made. The abdominal incision should be at least 20 cm long and the viscera should be carefully examined. Most liver, and some splenic, ruptures can be managed by suture. Rupture of the pancreas, usually in the midline, should be treated by distal pancreatectomy with ligation of the proximal pancreatic duct and lesser sac drainage. Rupture of the posterior wall of the duodenum can easily, and fatally, be overlooked. Rupture of jejunum or ileum should usually be treated by resection and anastomosis. Provided laparotomy is carried out within approximately 6 hours of injury, before bacterial peritonitis has been established, no more than two more doses of antibiotic need be given.

Infections following severe chest and head injuries

Whereas the maintenance of arterial oxygenation on the one hand, and the early diagnosis and treatment of cerebral compression on the other hand, are of paramount importance, it is essential to safeguard these patients against infections in the lungs, blood-stream (as a result of vascular devices), urinary tract and meninges. All these infections are hospital-acquired, and they are all potentially lethal. Avoidance of sputum retention and strict attention to all aspects of asepsis are far more important than administration of antibiotics, which should be reserved for the treatment of microbiologically-proven infections. It is, however, customary in most neurosurgical centres, although the custom is unsupported by the evidence of random control clinical trials, to give prophylactic sulphonamides or antibiotics or both to patients with basal skull fractures causing external leakage of cerebrospinal fluid.[3] The danger of meningitis is of such paramount concern that none of these centres is willing to question such a regimen.

References

1. Gustilo RB, Anderson JT. Prevention of infection in the treatment of 1025 open fractures of long bones: retrospective and prospective analyses. *J Bone Joint Surg* 1976; **58A**:453–458.
2. Evans C, Rashid A, Rosenberg IL, Pollock AV. An appraisal of peritoneal lavage in the diagnosis of the acute abdomen. *Br J Surg* 1975; **62**:119–120.
3. Ignelzi RJ, van der Ark GD. Analysis of the treatment of basilar skull fractures with and without antibiotics. *J Neurosurg* 1975; **43**:721–725.

14

Infections following penetrating injuries

Any break in the skin or mucous membranes can allow the invasion of bacteria which, if they are of sufficient virulence to overcome the local and systemic host defences, will multiply and cause infection. Apart from the occasional perforation of the respiratory or gastro-intestinal tract by inhaled or swallowed foreign bodies, these injuries are the result of external violence.

The amount of tissue destruction, which is one of the most important causes of failure of the host to respond to bacterial invasion, depends on the kinetic energy of the penetrating object. This is proportional to the mass of the object and the square of its velocity. It is therefore obvious that a stab wound is less dangerous than a low-velocity hand-gun wound and that the most dangerous injury is caused by a high-velocity bullet, or shrapnel, which expend nearly all their kinetic energy in widespread destruction of the tissues which lie in their path. The outlook for abdominal penetrating wounds depends on the age of the patient, the presence or absence of left colon injury, the number of organs injured, and the amount of blood required to achieve haemodynamic stability. These were the significant risk factors identified by stepwise logistic regression in 145 patients by Nichols and his colleagues who found that infections complicated 23 out of 101 gunshot wounds and 4 out of 41 stab wounds.[1] The 95 per cent confidence limits for relative risk were 0.88–8.46, indicating that too few patients were included to allow acceptance of the null hypothesis that the two causes of injury were equally dangerous.

Knives are relatively, and bullets absolutely, sterile; bacteria originate from the patient's clothing or skin, from the soil in cases of bomb explosions and from the contents of perforated hollow viscera. Human and animal bites are special cases in that the instrument itself is infected.

Human and animal bites

These present special problems. Not only are the tissues likely to be severely traumatized and devascularized, but also the teeth, and particularly the plaques which form on ill-tended human teeth, are heavily infected with both aerobic and anaerobic organisms. Extra care must therefore be taken to excise damaged skin and deeper tissues after administering a single dose of an antibiotic; oral anaerobes are sensitive to the penicillins and cephalosporins. Saline lavage, unless under high pressure, is useless but scrubbing the wound with chlorhexidine detergent and water will help remove particulate contamination.[2] Facial and upper limb bites may then be sutured, but bites on the trunk or lower limbs are best left for delayed suture or to heal by granulation.

Rabies

Rabies does not exist in Britain, but in countries where it is endemic it is desirable to secure, isolate and observe any animal which has bitten a person. If the animal shows symptoms of rabies it should be killed and the brain examined for Negri bodies. If it is a wild animal such as a fox or wolf, and the attack was unprovoked, the animal should be regarded as rabid.

Untreated, rabies is uniformly fatal and, if there is a high degree of suspicion, it is necessary to undertake immediate prophylaxis by local and intramuscular injection of 20 IU/kg of human hyperimmune globulin together with 1 ml of killed human diploid cell rabies vaccine, the latter to be repeated on days 3, 7, 14 and 28. Untoward reactions to this regimen are uncommon.

Stab wounds

Apart from minimal excision of the skin edges and primary closure of wounds seen within 6 hours, surgical intervention is necessary only if there is evidence of uncontrolled internal bleeding or of perforation of a hollow viscus. These patients should be given a single dose of an antibiotic when they are first seen, and then the wound should be excised and closed and the patient kept under observation. Formal laparotomy or thoracotomy should only be undertaken if the vital signs, notably the state of peripheral perfusion, the pulse and the blood pressure, show deterioration.

Low-velocity missile wounds

In countries where the possession of hand-guns is legal the treatment of these wounds occupies a great deal of surgical time. In the USA it has been estimated that more than 20 000 people died of bullet wounds in 1981.[3]

The kinetic energy released by a hand-gun bullet is much greater than that of a stab and much less than that of a high-velocity missile. The corollary is that, unlike patients with stab wounds, these patients should undergo formal exploration under general anaesthesia after resuscitation. They should be given an antibiotic intravenously as soon as possible after the injury; the choice of a beta-lactamase-resistant penicillin or a cephalosporin or an aminoglycoside, with or without metronidazole, depends on the internal organs suspected of being injured. Devitalized tissue must be excised and perforations of hollow viscera closed or, in the case of the left colon, exteriorized. The skin may be closed if operation is undertaken within approximately 6 hours of the injury; if operation has to be delayed for any reason, the skin should not be sutured. When dealing with gross peritoneal contamination from colonic perforations some surgeons do not even close the aponeurosis primarily, but use a sheet of Silastic, Marlex or polytetrafluoroethylene (Gore-tex) to retain the intestines for the first 5 days and either suture the aponeurosis at a second operation after that time or leave the wound to heal by granulation.

High-velocity missile wounds

Rifle bullets and fragments of exploding shells and bombs are the main causes of injuries in war-time, including terrorist attacks. Apart from the rules which apply to all wounds – immediate staunching of major haemorrhage, securing a clear airway, early intravenous antibiotic administration and correction of hypovolaemia – there are three special aspects of the operative treatment of these patients.

First, when there are dozens of casualties, the surgeon must decide on whom to operate first: this demands triage – the grading of severity and probable outcome. Secondly, because the amount of kinetic energy released is much greater, there is more internal damage than would appear from the appearance of the skin wound, and extensive excision of devitalized tissue is necessary. Finally, the skin should not be closed primarily but the wound should be covered with a sterile dressing and either closed secondarily or the granulation tissue grafted.

Tetanus and gas gangrene

The clostridia which cause these potentially lethal complications are widely distributed, particularly in manured soil. Even a mere scratch may allow the entrance of *Clostridium tetani* which, if it multiplies, produces an exotoxin which causes tetanus in non-immune subjects. Tetanus is unknown when a population is protected by active immunization with tetanus toxoid. The organism is sensitive to penicillin, and patients with even trivial wounds which may have been contaminated by cultivated soil should be given a prophylactic dose of penicillin and a booster dose of tetanus toxoid. In Third World countries neonatal tetanus is a major cause of death, and it is only by active immunization of the whole population that such waste can be avoided.[4]

Treatment of tetanus

Tetanus is common in the islands of the South Pacific. Phillips published a classification of tetanus,[5] allocating scores both to the initial severity of the attack (Table 14.1) and to the response to treatment (Table 14.2). An initial score of 24 or more indicates severe disease with death as the expected outcome; 15–23 is severe with survival depending on the quality of treatment. A patient with a score of 10–14 should survive with any reasonable standard of care, and below 10 spontaneous recovery is to be expected.

Ahmadsyah and Salim in Jakarta treated 172 patients with moderate tetanus (Phillips score 9–19) by excision of wounds, daily intramuscular tetanus antitoxin for 5 days and heavy sedation.[6] Oxygen was given and a tracheostomy was performed if necessary. In addition the patients were allocated, but not randomized, to receive either procaine penicillin 1.5 mU intramuscularly 8-hourly for 7–10 days or metronidazole 500 mg orally

Table 14.1 Factors determining severity of tetanus

Factor	Score
Incubation time	
less than 48 hours	5
2–5 days	4
5–10 days	3
10–14 days	2
more than 14 days	1
Site of infection	
internal and umbilical	5
head, neck and body wall	4
peripheral proximal	3
peripheral distal	2
unknown	1
State of protection	
none	10
possibly some or neonate's mother immunized	8
protected more than 10 years ago	4
protected less than 10 years ago	2
'complete' protection	0
Complicating factors	
injury or illness hazarding life, or neonate	10
severe injury or illness not immediately hazarding life	8
injury or illness not hazarding life	4
minor injury or illness	2
ASA grade 1	0

Adapted from Phillips LA. A classification of tetanus. *Lancet* 1967; **i**: 1216–17 by kind permission of the publishers.

6-hourly or 1 g rectally 8-hourly for 7–10 days. Eighteen of the 76 patients given penicillin died, compared with seven of the 97 patients given metronidazole ($P = 0.005$). Hospital stay was, on average, 5 days shorter in the metronidazole group.

Gas gangrene

Gas gangrene is usually caused by *Clostridium perfringens*, which is a common inhabitant of the colon, although other clostridia and, particularly in diabetics, non-clostridial organisms may cause it. *Cl. perfringens* cannot start multiplying in an aerobic environment, but if it takes hold in dead tissue it can then spread rapidly to previously well-vascularized parts, causing death of the tissues, severe pain and toxaemia. Treatment is by penicillin together with immediate radical excision of all gangrenous skin, muscle and fascia; in the lower limb this usually implies high amputation without skin closure. Although gas gangrene used to be common in wounded soldiers, it is now more often seen in civilian practice. Early antibiotic administration, careful debridement of devitalized tissue and avoidance of primary skin closure are the main principles of prophylaxis.

Table 14.2 Factors determining the course of an attack of tetanus

Factor	Score
Severity of spasms	
opisthotonos	5
whole-body spasms	4
limited spasms	3
generalized stiffness	2
trismus only	1
Frequency of spasms	
3 or more spontaneous in 15 minutes	5
less than 3 spontaneous in 15 minutes	4
occasional spontaneous	3
with stimuli only	2
less than 6 in 12 hours	1
Body temperature (°C)	
under 36.7 or over 38.9	10
38.3–38.8	8
37.8–38.2	4
37.2–37.7	2
36.7–37.1	0
Respiration	
tracheostomy	10
apnoeic after all spasms	8
apnoeic after the occasional spasm	4
apnoeic during spasms only	2
minimal interference	0

Adapted from Phillips LA. A classification of tetanus. *Lancet* 1967; **i**: 1216–17 by kind permission of the publishers.

References

1. Nichols RL, Smith JW, Klein DB, Trunkey DD, Cooper RH, Adinolfi MF, Mills J. Risk of infection after penetrating abdominal trauma. *New Eng J Med* 1984; **311**:1065–1070.
2. Madden J, Edlich RF, Schauerhamer R, Prusak M, Borner J, Wangensteen OH. Application of principles of fluid dynamics to surgical wound irrigation. *Cur Top Surg Res* 1971; **3**:85–93.
3. Schetky DH. Children and handguns. A public health concern. *Am J Dis Child* 1985; **139**:229–231.
4. World Health Organization Weekly Epidemiological Record 1985; **60**:227–229.
5. Phillips LA. A classification of tetanus. *Lancet* 1967; **i**:1216–1217.
6. Ahmadsyah I, Salim A. Treatment of tetanus: an open study to compare the efficacy of procaine penicillin and metronidazole. *Brit Med J* 1985; **291**:648–650.

15

Infections of the skin and subcutaneous tissues

The skin is a highly efficient antimicrobial barrier. It harbours a large resident population of bacteria, mainly coagulase-negative staphylococci and corynebacteria, and is frequently, but temporarily, colonized by other organisms which do no harm provided there is no break in the integrity of the barrier and provided the ducts of the skin, sweat, sebaceous and apocrine glands remain patent. Very few of these infections require surgical attention, and I am going to restrict myself to consideration of three acute (cellulitis, abscess and infective gangrene) and three chronic infections (ulcers, sinuses and recurrent hydradenitis suppurativa).

Cellulitis

Although this is classically the result of invasion by *Streptococcus pyogenes* of Lancefield group A through what may have been an unperceived break in the skin barrier, it may also be caused by numerous other organisms, particularly if host defences are reduced locally by ischaemia or generally by malnutrition, uncontrolled diabetes or immune deficiency syndromes.

Cellulitis must be distinguished, not only from the various forms of infective gangrene, but also from the purely cutaneous infection of erysipelas and from two skin manifestations of distant *Staphylococcus aureus* infection. These are the staphylococcal scalded skin syndrome of infants, usually the result of umbilical infection,[1] and the toxic shock syndrome of adults, usually the result of vaginal infection associated with tampons.[2] In the former an epidermolysin and, in the latter, exotoxin C and enterotoxin F are implicated. Prophylaxis in infants is by sterilization of the umbilicus with an antiseptic such as 70 per cent isopropyl alcohol or 0.33 per cent hexachlorophane powder, and in adults by frequent changes of tampons or avoidance of their use.

Antibiotic treatment of cellulitis is indicated, initially by penicillin G parenterally, but every effort must be made to identify the bacterial cause and to select the most appropriate drug. Examination of swabs from an apparent site of entry is usually misleading, but two reliable techniques are available. Injection and aspiration of 1 ml of sterile saline into the area of cellulitis followed by Gram-staining and culture of the fluid may allow accurate identification of the causative organisms. Alternatively, Pruitt advocates biopsy under local anaesthesia with examination of a Gram-stained frozen section of part of the specimen, and culture of the rest.[3] This method is particularly valuable in differentiating cellulitis, correctly treated by anti-biotics alone, from necrotizing fasciitis which demands wide surgical excision.[4]

Abscess

An abscess implies that the body defences have successfully contained invading bacteria, but complete resolution depends on evacuation of the pus and obliteration of the cavity.

The traditional and widely used treatment is by incision and drainage under antibiotic cover, with or without excision of skin on the apex of the abscess – a technique designed to prevent premature skin healing. This method, essential for most infections in the hand, has, however, several disadvantages including pain, frequent dressings, and delay in both healing and return to work. The alternative, which achieves primary healing in a high proportion of cases, is to incise the abscess and use a blunt curette or a gloved finger to evacuate all pus, foreign bodies and slough. The edges of the skin incision may be allowed to fall together or they may be drawn together with adhesive tapes. This technique was introduced 30 years ago and was thought to require pre-operative administration of an antibiotic for its success. Recently, however, a similar success rate has been achieved without the use of an antibiotic.[6] In the perianal region, if an abscess is associated with an anal fistula, permanent healing will be achieved only after cure of the fistula.

It is always advisable to send pus for microbiological examination. Although the most commonly isolated bacterium is *Staph. aureus*, many other aerobic and anaerobic organisms may cause abscesses. Failure of an incised abscess to heal may indicate an unrecognized intestinal fistula, a retained slough or foreign body or, rarely, a specific infection, for example by *Mycobacterium tuberculosis* or *Actinomyces israelii*. These conditions are to be sought by microscopic examination of biopsy material and special culture techniques, and then require specific antimicrobial chemotherapy.

Infections around the anus

Peri-anal and ischiorectal abscesses are among the most common of all subcutaneous abscesses which present to the general surgeon. They arise in one of two ways. *Staph. aureus* can cause infection of the skin glands here as in any other part of the body. These have no connection with the anal canal and heal permanently after incision or spontaneous drainage.

The number of these infections is, however, far exceeded by those abscesses which arise from infection in the anal glands, which are at the level of the anal crypts at the dentate line, halfway up the anal canal. Some anal glands lie deep to the internal anal sphincter muscle (the continuation of the inner circular layer of smooth muscle of the rectum), and infection arising from invasion of faecal aerobic and anaerobic bacteria may cause an abscess between the internal and external sphincter. From here the abscess expands to present in the subcutaneous tissue of the peri-anal region, its inner boundary being the internal sphincter. Occasionally, however, it spreads up and down in the intersphincteric space, causing great pain but without visible external signs of an abscess. On the other hand, a few of these abscesses traverse the external sphincter and then present in the ischiorectal fossa. For some reason which is not clear, such penetration occurs only if the primary infection is in an anal gland in the posterior midline.

Anal gland abscesses which are confined externally by the internal sphincter heal after discharging into the anal canal. Those which penetrate the internal sphincter usually present as peri-anal abscesses and, if they also discharge into the anal canal, external drainage of the abscess is likely to leave a low level anal fistula. Those rare abscesses which extend through the external sphincter muscle complex are likely to spread bilaterally in the fatty ischiorectal fossa and lead to a 'horse-shoe' fistula with an internal opening in the posterior midline of the anal canal. Suprasphincteric abscesses and fistulae are uncommon and arise either in association with rectal diseases like Crohn's, or as a result of overenthusiastic excision of a high anal fistula.

Treatment

I am astonished at the number of peri-anal and even ischiorectal abscesses which are sent to a surgeon after several days treatment with antibiotics – and usually the wrong antibiotic (e.g. flucloxacillin). Patients with peri-anal suppuration are surgical emergencies. Following a single dose of metro-nidazole 500 mg intravenously together with a cephalosporin or amino-glycoside, operation must be undertaken. The classical incision is a cruciate one, excising enough skin to allow free drainage. I prefer, however, a linear incision, careful debridement of the cavity and then a simple dry dressing. A finger in the anal canal will sometimes identify an internal opening and, if this is obvious, the intervening tissue between the external incision and the internal opening should be incised and some skin sacrificed to produce a wound which can heal by granulation. Surgical treatment of high anal fistulae requires above all the accurate identification of the internal opening, together with the discovery and unroofing of all the ramifications in the ischiorectal fossa. A true rectocutaneous fistula associated with Crohn's or other rectal disease is usually an indication for elective proctectomy.

Pilonidal abscess and sinus

Hairs can penetrate the skin of the gluteal cleft and allow the entrance of bacteria which can cause an abscess. Spontaneous or operative evacuation of the pus leaves a sinus leading to a cavity lined by granulation tissue and containing loose hairs. It often has side tracks into one or both buttocks. The condition is common in young men and, even in the absence of definitive treatment, practically never persists after the age of 40 years. The treatment should be as conservative as possible – an abscess should be incised and hairs removed, whereas a relatively symptomless sinus can usually be successfully managed by instructing the patient to brush the gluteal cleft with a tooth brush during his daily bath. Sinuses causing significant symptoms or recur-rent abscesses need operation, but there is no evidence that radical excision with or without primary suture is any more effective than conservative laying open of the tracks, allowing healing by second intention. Antibiotics play no part in treatment.

Inflammation of salivary glands

Community-acquired sialitis usually involves the submaxillary salivary glands, where it complicates ductal obstruction by a concretion. It responds to antibiotic treatment but recurrence can only be prevented by sialectomy. Acute parotitis, apart from that caused by mumps virus, is almost always caused by invasion by alpha- or beta-haemolytic streptococci, with or without parotid duct obstruction and sialectasis. It responds to oral penicillin, and parotidectomy should only be undertaken in patients who are seriously inconvenienced by frequent recurrences. Occasionally, a parotid abscess may complicate bacterial parotitis and require incision. It is seldom followed by a salivary fistula but, if it is, again parotidectomy is indicated.

Postoperative parotitis used to be common in patients who suffered intra-abdominal complications after operations. It is now rare, possibly as a result of better knowledge of fluid requirements.

Infective gangrene

This is a dangerous condition. Infection may be secondary to gangrene, or gangrene may be secondary to infection.

Infection secondary to gangrene

Invasion of any pathogenic bacterium through a break in the skin of an ischaemic limb can cause gangrene. It is common, and becoming more common, as more people live long enough to suffer arteriosclerotic occlusion of lower limb vessels.

Initially, treatment requires bed-rest, analgesics and antibiotics. As the local circulation is precarious, it is inadvisable to try to make an accurate microbiological diagnosis of the infection by biopsy of the spreading cellulitis, and swabs from the surface of the gangrene seldom yield useful information. Antibiotics must therefore be prescribed without knowledge of the infecting organism and I would choose a second- or third-generation cephalosporin administered parenterally. If the patient is diabetic, he will usually require insulin until the infection is controlled.

The next step is to assess the possibility of reconstructive arterial surgery. Although newer, relatively non-invasive methods such as digital subtraction angiography and Doppler wave analysis may be helpful, a percutaneous arteriogram is usually essential. This will show occlusion of at least two main arteries, and the decision about an attempt to revascularize the limb will depend on the technical possibility of bypassing the occlusions, preferably with an autogenous reversed or, when the anastomosis is to be made to a tibial artery, *in situ* vein graft. If the arteriographic appearances indicate the impossibility of bypassing the occlusions, or if a bypass operation fails, then amputation is indicated. The site (transmetatarsal, below-knee or above-knee) must be judged clinically; diabetics heal lower amputations better than non-diabetics. The ultimate outcome is poor and few diabetic or non-diabetic patients are alive 5 years after developing gangrene.

Gangrene secondary to infection

When invading bacteria are of sufficient virulence to overwhelm local defences, one of two conditions results: rapidly spreading cellulitis and early bacterial invasion of lymphatics and blood-stream, or progressive gangrene of viable tissues. It is not only the aggressive nature of the organisms which is responsible for bacterial gangrene, but also the failure of the host to localize and destroy the invaders. This failure may be caused by general or local factors. General factors include malnutrition, iatrogenic interference with the immune system by steroids or cytotoxic chemotherapy, and severe trauma including anaesthesia and operations. The most important local factors are the presence of foreign bodies and crushed tissues.

Gas gangrene (clostridial myonecrosis)

This potentially lethal condition is nearly always caused by unopposed invasion of *Clostridium perfringens*, although other clostridia may occasionally be responsible. Strict adherence to the three principles of the treatment of missile injuries – immediate prophylactic antibiotic, early debridement and delayed skin closure – has practically eliminated gas gangrene in war wounds, but it is still seen occasionally in civilian practice after compound fractures, leg or thigh amputations for arteriosclerotic gangrene and perforations of the colon. It is characterized by severe pain, toxaemia (which may progress to multiple organ failure) and the presence of gas in the muscles and subcutaneous tissues. Urgent treatment with large doses of penicillin parenterally and excision of all involved tissues is necessary. The place of hyperbaric oxygen treatment has not been firmly established; it is in any case secondary to the absolute necessity of radical debridement, adequate antibiotic therapy and treatment of septic shock.

Septicaemic gangrene

Scattered areas of cutaneous gangrene may appear in patients with meningococcal or pseudomonas septicaemia. Such patients are severely ill and require resuscitation and parenteral antibiotics; excision and grafting of dead skin may be needed later.

Necrotizing fasciitis and progressive bacterial gangrene

These conditions comprise all cases of non-clostridial infective gangrene involving the subcutaneous tissue and skin. There are differences in the bacterial flora associated with different manifestations of the conditions, but they all have in common the failure of the body to localize and destroy aerobic and anaerobic bacteria. These bacteria proliferate, causing destruction in the subcutaneous and fascial planes; arterial and venous thrombosis leads to dermal gangrene.

Group A beta-haemolytic streptococci may cause the condition after minor trauma, Meleney's progressive synergistic gangrene is associated with a micro-aerophilic streptococcus, cancrum oris (noma) with fusiform and spirochaetal organisms, and Fournier's scrotal gangrene and postoperative necrotizing fasciitis of the abdominal wall with aerobic and anaerobic faecal organisms. Biopsy of the gangrenous tissue with Gram-staining and culture will usually identify the causative bacteria.[4]

The severity of the systemic symptoms varies; necrotizing fasciitis causes the most severe and often rapidly fatal toxaemia. Treatment by intravenous fluid administration, parenteral antibiotics and urgent wide excision of dead tissue, which extends much further than the limits of the dermal gangrene, are essential. Until a microbiological diagnosis is available, I prefer to administer an aminoglycoside with metronidazole. No attempt should be made to provide primary skin cover after debridement; the raw area should be covered by sterile dressings which are changed under general anaesthesia every other day. Secondary skin grafting must await resolution of the gangrene.

Ulcers

Although the term may correctly be used to describe any skin or mucosal defect, I will restrict my discussion to infected skin defects which have not healed after a month. I discuss full-thickness burns in Chapter 11.

Ischaemic ulcers

There are three conditions which lead to the supply of oxygenated blood being insufficient both to maintain skin integrity and to restore it if it is breached. These conditions are venous stasis, arterial occlusion and pressure. Bacteria play little initial part in their aetiology, although secondary bacterial invasion is common; this can lead to enlargement of the ulcer and may cause cellulitis or necrotizing fasciitis.

Venous stasis ulcers

Chronic venous stasis in the lower leg, associated with incompetent valves in superficial, deep and perforating veins, leads to extravasation of plasma which clots and overwhelms the local fibrinolytic mechanisms. The fibrin deposits are recognized clinically by hardening of the skin and loss of the ability to wrinkle it, the condition known as scleroedema or lipodermatosclerosis. The effect of these perivascular fibrin deposits is to deprive the skin of nourishment.[7] Secondary bacterial invasion sufficient to cause cellulitis may require systemic antibiotics, but topical antibiotics are contra-indicated for the same reasons as in full-thickness burns. The principles of treatment are compression bandaging, nocturnal elevation of the limb, avoidance of standing and encouragement to walk. Painful ulcers are best treated by excision through deep fascia followed by skin grafting, but compression and nocturnal elevation must be continued indefinitely. Fibrinolytic enhancement by stanozolol has shown promise in a controlled clinical trial.[8] The recommended dose is 10 mg/day by mouth.

Patients who are overweight or aged, and particularly those whose skin has atrophied as a result of long-continued steroid therapy, present great problems in treatment, and recurrent ulceration is common. The importance of compression bandaging cannot be overstressed. Wound dressings are of secondary importance, and I have yet to be convinced that any of the newer polymer dressings are superior to non-adherent gauze. In the treatment of ulcers of any type which are covered by slough, the polysaccharide dextranomer (Debrisan) or the disaccharide granulated sugar can achieve rapid debridement and formation of granulation tissue.[9]

Ulcers associated with arterial occlusion

Sudden unrelieved arterial occlusion of more than one major lower limb artery results in gangrene. Ischaemic ulceration, on the other hand, is the result of a break in the skin barrier of a chronically ischaemic foot or lower leg. These ulcers are usually painful and will not heal unless at least one of the occluded arteries can be bypassed by a vein graft below the inguinal ligament or a synthetic graft above the ligament. Secondary bacterial invasion is common, and antibiotics and debridement of dead tissue are an integral part of the treatment.

Pressure ulcers

If the skin is compressed against an underlying bone for more than about 3 hours, its blood supply may be permanently cut off, resulting in pressure necrosis. Discomfort is the normal stimulus for a person to move about in bed, and paraplegic patients are at special risk of developing bed sores. Comatose, paralysed and severely ill patients must be turned from side to side every hour, even when special mattresses are used.

The treatment of these ulcers is difficult. It is essential to avoid any further compression and then either to allow slow ingrowth of new epithelium from the edges of the ulcer, or to cover the defect with a full-thickness rotation flap. Antibiotics must be used only if the ulcer is complicated by cellulitis.

Malignant ulcers

The situation and appearance of the ulcer which has a rolled edge in basal cell carcinoma, a raised everted edge in squamous carcinoma, and traces of black pigment in melanoma, usually give away the diagnosis. Treatment is normally by wide excision with or without skin grafting, but some basal cell carcinomas and most ulcerating breast carcinomas are best treated by radiotherapy, combined in the latter case with tamoxifen or cytotoxic chemotherapy. Antibiotics play no part in the treatment, but the unpleasant odour of an ulcerating breast carcinoma can sometimes be controlled by topical application of metronidazole.

Ulcers caused by specific microorganisms

Although these ulcers are rare in western countries, surgeons should be alert to the possibility of syphilis in the form of a primary chancre or breaking-down gumma, tuberculosis, actinomycosis, anthrax, fuso-spirochaetal tropical ulcers, chlamydial lymphogranuloma venereum, calymmatobacterial granuloma inguinale, fungal Madura foot, cutaneous amoebiasis and leishmaniasis (oriental sore). Specific antimicrobial treatment is indicated for these conditions. In immunosuppressed patients, herpes simplex or zoster infections may cause extensive necrosis and ulceration.

Sinuses and fistulae

A sinus can be differentiated from an ulcer because its root cause is the presence of a foreign body in the deeper tissues. A sinus may heal from time to time, only to break out again in the form of an abscess which discharges to become once more a sinus. Permanent cure cannot be achieved until that foreign body is removed or, when the sinus is an intestinal fistula, the internal opening closes either spontaneously or as a result of surgery.

The nature of the bacteria associated with these conditions is relatively immaterial as far as treatment is concerned, but the presence of *Bacteroides fragilis* in the pus usually indicates that there is a connection with the intestine. Removal of the foreign body may be easy when, for example, it is the knot of a non-absorbable suture used for abdominal wall closure, or it may require an extensive operation when the foreign body is an infected arterial graft or a bone sequestrum. Removal of the hairs from a pilonidal sinus will allow healing, but there is a considerable tendency for the condition to recur when hairs are again thrust into the subcutaneous tissues.

A spontaneous intestinal fistula seldom heals until the internal opening is closed by resection of the diseased segment of bowel or, in the case of an anal fistula, until the track is laid open, allowing it to heal by granulation. Postoperative fistulae, on the other hand, have a strong tendency to heal provided the patient's nutritional requirements are properly met. It is in the treatment of small bowel fistulae that parenteral hyperalimentation has most firmly established its value.

Suppurative hidradenitis

Staphylococcal infection of the apocrine glands in the axilla, groin or perineum results in recurrent abscesses and sinuses, and permanent cure can be achieved only by excision of all the involved skin and subcutaneous tissue. Patients with this condition have often suffered years of antibiotic administration before being referred to a surgeon.

References

1. Dowsett EG. The staphylococcal scalded skin syndrome. *J Hosp Infect* 1984; 5:347–54.
2. Thomas D, Withington PS. Toxic shock syndrome: a review of the literature. *Ann Roy Coll Surg Engl* 1985; **67**:156–58.

3. Pruitt B. Biopsy diagnosis of surgical infections. *New Eng J Med* 1984; **310**:1737–38.
4. Stamenkovic I, Lew PD. Early recognition of potentially fatal necrotizing fasciitis. *New Eng J Med* 1984; **310**:1689–93.
5. Watson N. Antibiotic in hand infections. *Brit Med J* 1985; **290**:491–92.
6. Stewart MPM, Laing MR, Krukowski ZH. Treatment of acute abscesses by incision, curettage and primary suture without antibiotics. A controlled clinical trial. *Brit J Surg* 1985; **72**:66–7.
7. Browse NL. Venous ulceration. *Brit Med J* 1983; **286**:1920–22.
8. Burnand K, Clemenson G, Morland M, Jarrett PEM, Browse NL. Venous lipodermatosclerosis: treatment by fibrinolytic enhancement and elastic compression. *Brit Med J* 1980; **i**:7–11.
9. Trouillet JL, Chastre J, Fagon JY, Pierre J, Domart Y, Gibert C. Use of granulated sugar in treatment of open mediastinitis after cardiac surgery. *Lancet* 1985; **ii**:180–84.

16

Infections of the lungs and heart

Community-acquired infections within the thoracic cavity are not primarily the concern of surgeons, but surgical techniques are often required and may be crucial in determining the outcome of an infection.

Empyema thoracis

In pre-antibiotic days empyema was often encountered as a complication of lobar pneumonia caused by *Streptococcus pneumoniae*, especially in children. *Strep. pneumoniae* is now an uncommon cause; most cases are the result either of penetrating wounds or of rupture of pulmonary, mediastinal or subdiaphragmatic abscesses into the pleural cavity. The microbiology has also changed, and coagulase-positive staphylococci which are the commonest causes of lung abscesses and pyopneumothorax in infants, Gram-negative rods and anaerobes are more likely to be isolated, often in mixed culture.

Diagnosis

Examination of the chest of a pyrexial breathless patient will disclose stony dullness on one side and breath sounds will not be heard. Postero-anterior and lateral chest X-rays will show the presence of fluid which requires withdrawal by closed needle aspiration and immediate despatch to the laboratory for Gram-staining and aerobic and anaerobic culture. Only then should antibiotic treatment be started. Of equal importance is the detection of the cause of the empyema; a neighbouring abscess requires treatment at the same time as the empyema. Chest X-rays (after evacuating the pleural fluid), ultrasonography, computerized tomography, barium meal X-rays, oesophagoscopy and bronchoscopy may all be required.

Treatment

The patient requires urgent admission to hospital for daily needle thoracentesis and parenteral antibiotic treatment appropriate to the bacteria identified in the fluid. A causative abscess must be drained or excised. In most cases these measures are enough to ensure resolution, although closed drainage by an intercostal tube is often required. Occasionally, the lung fails to expand to fill the thoracic cavity, becoming encapsulated in a thick layer of fibrin and pyogenic membrane on both visceral and parietal pleura. This is an indication for late thoracotomy and decortication of the pleural surfaces, followed by closed suction drainage. Appropriate antibiotic treatment should be continued until the chest drain is removed. Chronic empyema is rare in patients who have received proper treatment early in the course of their disease, and there is little indication these days for operations such as thoracoplasty to obliterate a chronic abscess cavity in the pleura. Chronic empyema following pneumonectomy may, however, require thoracoplasty and drainage of the remaining space.

Lung abscess

Although the management of community-acquired acute infections in the lungs is almost exclusively non-surgical, the surgeon may occasionally be called upon to deal with a complicated lung abscess. Progression of primary pneumonia from consolidation to abscess formation is rare when antibiotics are prescribed, and lung abscesses are usually the result of inhalation of particulate matter, of bronchial obstruction by carcinoma or of septic embolization in immunocompromised patients. Anaerobic bacteria usually take part in the destruction of lung tissue, and this accounts for the foul smell of the sputum which these patients produce when the abscess breaks through into a bronchus.

Surgical expertise may be required both for diagnosis and for treatment. Accurate identification of the causative bacteria is essential in planning antibiotic therapy and an early diagnostic step is aerobic and anaerobic culture of the sputum, if necessary by percutaneous puncture of the trachea, injection of 1 ml of saline, and aspiration of the sputum which is generated. Bronchoscopy is essential to diagnose inhaled foreign bodies or bronchial neoplasms. The flexible fibre-optic bronchoscope is valuable for this purpose and can be introduced in the conscious patient. Transbronchial aspiration of an abscess can be dangerous, allowing spread of infection or even drowning if a massive quantity of pus is suddenly liberated.

Provided appropriate antibiotics, starting with penicillin after specimens have been obtained for culture, are prescribed for a reasonable length of time, surgical treatment is not required except for excision of a lobe or a lung for an abscess caused by an irremovable foreign body or a bronchial neoplasm. Transthoracic drainage of a lung abscess is not indicated.

Bronchiectasis

Forty years ago lobectomy for bronchiectasis was one of the most frequently performed thoracic operations. Antibiotics and physiotherapy have entirely changed the picture, and it is now rare for surgeons to be called on to deal with an unresponsive or recurrent case.[1]

Pulmonary tuberculosis

The introduction of streptomycin in 1945 revolutionized the treatment of pulmonary tuberculosis. Antibiotic-resistant strains soon emerged, and streptomycin is no longer the first-line drug; modern medical treatment is by the simultaneous oral administration of at least two of the other four effective drugs – isoniazid, ethambutol, pyrazinamide and rifampicin – for at least 1 year. There are now only two indications for operation, and only one appropriate operation – excision. The indications are, first, the discovery on a chest X-ray of a solitary non-cavitating non-calcified shadow, the nature of which can only be determined histologically. These tuberculomas look like bronchogenic carcinomas on X-ray and require excision. The second indication is the failure of adequate three-drug medical treatment to effect a clinical and radiographic cure. Such failure may be the result of the presence of drug-resistant organisms or of poor compliance on the part of the patient who may not understand the necessity for long-continued drug treatment.

Rare pulmonary infections which may simulate bronchogenic carcinoma

It is proper for surgeons to excise, by segmental resection, lobectomy or pneumonectomy, undiagnosed pulmonary lesions which resemble bronchogenic carcinomas on chest X-ray. Although the majority of these lesions will turn out to be cancers, there will be some which are found to be caused by atypical mycobacteria, actinomyces, histoplasma, coccidioides, aspergillus or cryptococcus. Hydatid cysts are a special case. They should be recognized on X-rays because of their clear-cut margins without surrounding shadowing. Medical treatment with albendazole, which is metabolized to the sulphoxide and in that form is capable of penetrating the cyst wall and killing the protoscolices shows promise,[2] but most hydatid cysts should be excised intact after sterilizing the contents by injecting formalin, hypertonic saline or povidone iodine.

Antibiotic prophylaxis of endocarditis

Patients with damaged or prosthetic heart valves, ventricular septal defects and patent ductus arteriosus undergoing operations which may cause bacteraemia must be protected against lodgement and growth of bacteria in the endocardium. The British Society for Antimicrobial Chemotherapy Working Party recommended that such patients undergoing dental operations should receive 3 g amoxycillin by mouth 1 hour before the operation, or 1 g intramuscularly immediately before, and 1 g orally 6 hours later.[3] For other operations with a potential for causing bacteraemia the Working Party recommended pre-operative parenteral amoxycillin 1 g together with gentamicin 120 mg. For patients known to be allergic to penicillin, the recommendations were either erythromycin 1.5 g orally 1 hour before and 6 hours later, or pre-operative intravenous vancomycin 1 g together with gentamicin 120 mg.

Surgical treatment for infective endocarditis

Although the treatment of bacterial endocarditis is primarily by long courses of antibiotics, mechanical failure – particularly of the aortic valve – may cause death from uncontrollable cardiac failure. It is in such cases that early prosthetic valve replacement while antibiotic administration continues offers the only chance of survival. Infection of a prosthetic valve requires that the valve be removed and replaced.

Surgical treatment of pericarditis

Serous pericardial effusions are best managed by repeated needle aspiration. Purulent pericarditis is rare and usually requires partial pericardectomy and drainage either externally or into the pleural cavity together with appropriate antibiotic therapy. Chronic constrictive pericarditis, possibly the end result of an acute viral infection, requires excision of the pericardium.

References

1. Oschner A. Bronchiectasis. A disappearing pulmonary lesion. *N Y State J Med* 1975; **75**:1683–1686.
2. Morris DL, Chinnery J, Giorgiou G, Colematis B, Stamatakis J, Hardcastle JD. Penetration of albendazole sulphoxide into hydatid cysts and its effect on *in vitro* cultures. *Brit J Surg* 1985; **72**:409.
3. British Society for Antimicrobial Chemotherapy Working Party. Prophylaxis for endocarditis. *Lancet* 1981; **2**:1323–1326.

17

Peritonitis

Community-acquired infections of the peritoneal cavity seldom occur in the absence of perforation of a diseased intra-abdominal viscus, but there are exceptions. I will consider postoperative peritonitis and intra-abdominal abscesses in Chapter 32.

Aetiology of peritonitis

Peritonitis arising without pre-existing abdominal disease

Primary bacterial peritonitis

In pre-antibiotic days primary pneumococcal infection was a common cause of peritonitis in children. It is now rare (possibly as a result of antibiotic prevention of pneumococcal bacteraemia), and primary bacterial peritonitis occurs more often as a complication of ascites in patients who are already ill and lack proper immune competence as a result of cirrhosis or nephritis. In these cases peritonitis is more likely to be associated with aerobic intestinal bacteria than with Gram-positive organisms.[1] The presence of anaerobic bacteria nearly always implies the perforation of a viscus.

Peritonitis following abdominal trauma

Both penetrating and blunt abdominal injuries may cause peritonitis after breaches in the walls of hollow viscera. In the upper abdomen the peritonitis is usually chemical from leakage of gastric, duodenal, biliary or pancreatic fluid, but the resulting paralytic ileus allows ileal aerobic and anaerobic organisms access to the upper gastro-intestinal tract, and bacterial contamination of the peritoneum occurs within a few hours. Perforations of the ileum, colon and rectum cause immediate particulate and bacterial contamination. Peritonitis may be delayed for a day or two if the injury has caused separation from the intestine of the mesentery or mesocolon, resulting in intestinal infarction and secondary perforation.

Tuberculous peritonitis

This is rare except in developing countries where it is a common cause of ascites. Menzies and his colleagues reported a series of 98 patients who presented with ascites in Lesotho;[2] laparoscopy, with or without biopsy, showed the presence of tuberculous peritonitis in 35 patients. The treatment is by oral administration for 9–12 months of at least two of the following drugs: ethambutol, rifampicin, isoniazid, para-amino salicylic acid, pyrazinamide.

Peritonitis following perforation of a diseased organ

Perforated peptic ulcer

The initial peritonitis is chemical; bacterial invasion becomes a threat only if treatment is delayed or is inefficient.

Pancreatitis

Here again the peritoneal inflammation is caused by the release of digestive enzymes. Bacterial contamination is rare in patients treated conservatively, but it may follow laparotomy whether or not the biliary tract is opened.

Biliary peritonitis

It is unusual for an inflamed or gangrenous gall bladder to perforate freely into the peritoneal cavity, more commonly it is isolated by omentum and neighbouring organs leading to an abscess or, occasionally, an enteric fistula. Free perforation carries a high mortality rate.[3]

Intestinal gangrene

Embolic occlusion of the superior mesenteric artery (usually associated with atrial fibrillation) or thrombosis of mesenteric arteries or veins, rapidly causes death of the part of the intestine supplied. There are, however, occasions when intestinal gangrene occurs without detectable vascular occlusion. Such an occurrence may be associated with an episode of hypovolaemic shock. The condition is both common and lethal in old people. The classical sign of abdominal rigidity is absent in the early stages, even though the patient is in great pain, and delay in laparotomy is almost always fatal.

Perforation of small bowel lesions

Many ulcerating and ischaemic lesions of the small intestine may perforate and cause bacterial peritonitis. They include ulcers secondary to ingested fish or chicken bones or impacted gall stones, Crohn's disease, Meckel's diverticulitis – usually associated with heterotopic gastric mucosa in the diverticulum – and, in tropical countries, typhoid fever. Strangulation of intestine as a result of internal hernia or volvulus round a band or adhesion will, if unrelieved, lead to perforation and peritonitis. Strangulated intestinal obstruction should never be neglected long enough for gangrene and perforation to occur.

Perforation of the appendix

This is probably the most frequent cause of peritonitis in Western countries. The polymicrobial infection which results from perforation of a gangrenous appendix is more often local than general. In a personal consecutive series of 251 patients operated on for perforated appendicitis, 148 infections were localized and 103 were generalized.

Perforation of large bowel lesions

Any ulcerating or ischaemic lesion of the colon may perforate, the extent of the resultant peritonitis depending on the size of the perforation, the rapidity of its development and the efficiency of host defences. A small slow perforation may lead to adherence of the bowel to neighbouring structures and, possibly, the formation of an enteric or vesical fistula. If the perforation is larger, an abscess may form. Potentially more lethal is the large free perforation of a stercoral or diverticular ulcer resulting in faecal contamination of the whole peritoneal cavity. Equally dangerous, but less common, are caecal perforations from unrelieved complete colonic obstruction, and the disintegration of the colon which may follow toxic megacolon in inflammatory bowel disease.

Diagnosis of peritonitis

Abdominal pain, vomiting and cessation of intestinal function are the cardinal symptoms of peritonitis. Examination shows a patient who is ill and dehydrated, and whose abdomen is tender and rigid. The temperature and pulse rate are raised and a blood count shows a neutrophil leucocytosis. Abdominal X-rays are of limited value; occasionally they may show gas under the diaphragm and frequently multiple fluid levels as a result of ileus. There are many atypical presentations, and it is for such patients that I have found the technique of diagnostic peritoneal lavage useful.[4]

Diagnostic peritoneal lavage

The abdominal wall in the midline near the umbilicus is infiltrated with local anaesthetic, avoiding any previous laparotomy scar. A plastic cannula is introduced into the peritoneal cavity and any free fluid aspirated; there is no need to continue with the lavage if fluid can be aspirated. The cannula is then connected to a 1-litre bag of sterile normal saline which is run in quickly, allowed to remain for 5 minutes and then to drain out by gravity. The most important test to make on the effluent is the examination of a stained film. If this shows a ratio of red cells to nucleated cells of less than 10:1, the diagnosis of local or general peritonitis can be made with confidence and laparotomy advised. Of secondary importance are culture of the fluid and estimation of amylase content; the latter may, however, be misleading – a high amylase content is often found in patients with intestinal strangulation.

Treatment of peritonitis

Replacement of fluid sequestered into the peritoneal cavity and intestines, removal of the source of bacterial contamination, and administration of appropriate antibacterial drugs are the cornerstones of treatment.

Many questions, however, still remain. What intravenous fluid and how much? What is the place of peroperative peritoneal lavage and postoperative dialysis with or without antibiotics? Is an intestinal anastomosis contra-indicated? Should the peritoneal cavity be drained? Should the skin be closed? What antibiotic should be given, by what route and for how long? These questions can best be answered by random control clinical trials, but the prognosis of peritonitis is so variable that some form of grading of severity is necessary if like is to be compared with like. Dellinger and his colleagues observed that published reports of trials of antibiotic treatment of intra-abdominal infections usually show a much lower mortality rate than audits of consecutive patients.[5]

I have discussed the principles of sepsis scoring in Chapter 7. These principles are applicable to peritonitis, but its cause must also be taken into account. The prognosis of chemical peritonitis from acute pancreatitis or perforation of a peptic ulcer depends not on the peritonitis *per se*, but on the extent of pancreatic necrosis in the former, and the timeliness and efficiency of operative repair of the perforation in the latter. As for bacterial peritonitis, that which is the result of perforation of the appendix is far less likely to be lethal than the peritonitis which follows intestinal gangrene or colonic perforation. It is clear that random control clinical trials of treatments for peritonitis must not mix all causes, but must stratify patients into groups with similar prognoses.

Intravenous fluid replacement

The surface area of the peritoneum is approximately 1.7 m^2 (roughly the same as that of the skin). When it is inflamed fluid is poured out; this rapidly depletes the volume of circulating blood. It is the loss of water and electrolytes which demands replacement by intravenous fluid. In an adult, 1 litre of normal saline or Hartmann's solution should be given in the first hour, the rate of infusion subsequently being monitored by clinical observations, by measurement of the central venous or pulmonary capillary wedge pressure and by the volume of urine output. Absorption of chemical or bacterial toxins from the peritoneum results in generalized capillary permeability and sequestration of fluid in the extravascular space. I found that fluid sequestration is one of the best guides to prognosis in acute pancreatitis.[6] In severe pancreatitis, defined by death or major complications, there was a discrepancy between the daily volume of fluid excreted in urine and gastric aspirate, and the amount infused, of more than 2 litres. This continued for at least 3 days or until death.

Therapeutic peritoneal lavage and dialysis

Peroperative lavage of a contaminated peritoneal cavity with several litres of normal saline, with or without the addition of an antibiotic or an antiseptic, is accepted without question by many surgeons.[7] No random control clinical trial has provided convincing evidence of its efficacy, and there are theoretical reasons to believe that it depletes humoral and cellular components of the host defences at the same time as it washes away bacteria.[8, 9] Antiseptics, even the newer, relatively non-toxic ones like chlorhexidine, povidone iodine and noxythcolin, cause as much damage to the host's cells as they do to bacterial.[10]

McAvinshey and his colleagues caused bacterial peritonitis in rats and found that noxythcolin peritoneal lavage did not increase the survival rate and that povidone iodine lavage reduced it.[11] Intramuscular amikacin together with metronidazole lavage reduced the mortality rate to zero.

Postoperative continuous peritoneal dialysis with a balanced electrolyte solution containing ampicillin 1 g/litre for 20 hours or a combination of gentamicin, cephalothin and lincomycin for 72 hours has been claimed to lower the rates of both sepsis and mortality, but the evidence is derived from non-randomized studies and is therefore subject to bias and error.[12, 13]

Intestinal anastomosis in the presence of peritonitis

The integrity of an intestinal anastomosis depends for the first few days on the sutures or staples which have been used, microscopic leaks being sealed by fibrin. Thereafter the healing process involves digestion of old collagen and laying down of new collagen. Bacteria produce enzymes capable of digesting both fibrin and collagen, and it is not safe to anastomose intestine in the presence of diffuse bacterial peritonitis. It is far better to resect the perforation or gangrene and exteriorize the bowel.

Drainage of the peritoneal cavity

As long ago as 1908, Yates came to the conclusion that 'the relative encapsulation of a drain is immediate. The absolute encapsulation occurs early (less than six hours in dogs)'.[14] There is no indication for drainage in patients with diffuse peritonitis.

Skin closure

The skin may safely be closed after laparotomy for chemical peritonitis from perforation of a peptic ulcer. After removal of a perforated appendix through a grid-iron incision it is wise to leave the skin open, either to heal by granulation or to be closed secondarily. Before embarking on secondary suture it is wise to make sure that the bacterial count is less than 10^5/g tissue. An open wound needs only dry dressings and heals in 1 month with a linear scar.[15] In a personal series of 96 perforated appendices treated in this way the median duration of hospital stay was 5.5 days and 86 per cent of patients stayed less than 10 days. Vertical laparotomy incisions do not heal as well as transverse incisions if the skin is left open but, in the presence of gross parietal contamination in operations for faecal peritonitis, the omission of skin sutures will usually avoid major aerobic and anaerobic wound infections. In patients with advanced peritonitis and multiple abscesses, particularly in association with anastomotic dehiscences and pancreatic necrosis, there is a place for non-closure of the aponeuroses as well as the skin.[16, 17]

I have not yet made up my mind about the place of polymethylmethacrylate beads incorporating gentamicin which are left in the sutured wound for 5 days. I have used these in 45 patients with peritonitis from perforation of the appendix and in 28 patients with peritonitis from perforation of the colon. Wound infections occurred in 19 patients (26 per cent) but only 6 (8 per cent) were associated with pyrexia and delayed the patient's discharge from hospital.

Antibiotics in the treatment of peritonitis

Peritonitis from perforation of a peptic ulcer of stomach or duodenum is sterile unless the operation has been delayed, and no more than a single pre-operative parenteral dose of a broad-spectrum anti-aerobic antibiotic is required for prophylaxis of infection. Nearly all bacterial peritonitis, on the other hand, is polymicrobial. Immediate incubation of pus in aerobic and anaerobic media will normally reveal coliforms, aerobic and anaerobic streptococci and *Bacteroides* species, mainly *Bacteroides fragilis*. This must be taken into account when choosing antibiotics for treatment, which should start before operation. Random control clinical trials have not helped much in making a choice, mainly because of lack of stratification for the severity of the infection.[5] Microbiological considerations prompt the use of an aminoglycoside to control coliforms, a penicillin for streptococci, and metronidazole, which is preferable to clindamycin both for effectiveness and lack of toxicity, for *B. fragilis*. It is traditional to continue the antibiotics for 5 days, but the duration of treatment should be determined by the clinical response of the patient rather than by any arbitrary figure.

References

1. Crossley IR, Williams R. Spontaneous bacterial peritonitis. *Gut* 1985; **26**:325–31.
2. Menzies RI, Fitzgerald JM, Mulpeter K. Laparoscopic diagnosis of ascites in Lesotho. *Brit Med J* 1985; **291**:473–75.
3. Harland C, Mayberry JF, Toghill PJ. Type 1 free perforation of the gallbladder. *J Roy Soc Med* 1985; **78**:725–28.
4. Evans C, Rashid A, Rosenberg IL, Pollock AV. An appraisal of peritoneal lavage in the diagnosis of the acute abdomen. *Brit J Surg* 1975; **62**:119–20.
5. Dellinger EP, Wertz MJ, Meakins JL, Solomkin JS, Allo MD, Howard RJ, Simmons RL. Surgical infection stratification system for intra-abdominal infection. Multicenter trial. *Arch Surg* 1985; **120**:21–29.
6. Sauven, P, Playforth MJ, Evans M, Pollock AV. Fluid sequestration: an early indicator of mortality in acute pancreatitis. *Brit J Surg* 1986; **73**:799–800.
7. Krukowski ZH, Stewart MPM, Alsasyer HM, Matheson NA. Infection after abdominal surgery: five year prospective study. *Brit Med J* 1984; **288**:278–280.
8. Nyström P-O, Skau T. Elimination patterns of *Escherichia coli* and *Bacteroides fragilis* from the peritoneal cavity. Studies with experimental peritonitis in pigs. *Acta Chir Scand* 1983; **149**:383–88.
9. Michel J, Bercovici B, Sacks T. Comparative studies on the antimicrobial activity

of peritoneal and ascitic fluid in human beings. *Surg Gynec Obstet* 1980; **151**:55–57.

10. Brennan SS, Leaper DJ. The effect of antiseptics on the healing wound: a study using the rabbit ear chamber. *Brit J Surg* 1985; **72**:780–782.

11. McAvinchey DJ, McCollum PT, Lynch G. Towards a rational approach to the treatment of peritonitis: an experimental study in rats. *Brit J Surg* 1984; **71**:715–17.

12. Normann E, Korvald E, Lotveit T. Perforated appendicitis – lavage or drainage? *Ann Chir Gyn Fenn* 1975; **64**:195–97.

13. Stephen M, Loewenthal J. Continuing peritoneal lavage in high-risk peritonitis. *Surgery* 1979; **85**:603–606.

14. Yates JL. An experimental study on the local effects of peritoneal drainage. *Surg Gynec Obstet* 1905; **1**:473–92.

15. Brennan SS, Smith GMR, Evans M, Pollock AV. The management of the perforated appendix: a controlled clinical trial. *Brit J Surg* 1982; **69**:510–12.

16. Maetani S, Tobe T. Open peritoneal drainage as effective treatment of advanced peritonitis. Surgery 1981; **90**:804–09.

17. Mughal MM, Bancewicz J, Irving MH. 'Laparostomy': a technique for the management of intractable intra-abdominal sepsis. *Brit J Surg* 1986; **73**:253–59.

18

Peptic ulcer and perforation

Aetiology

Peptic ulcers are caused by enzymatic digestion of gastric or duodenal walls, the innate resistance to acid-pepsin of which has been reduced. A species of campylobacter (*C. pyloridis*) has been detected microscopically in association with gastritis and peptic ulcer, and has recently been cultured, but its aetiological significance is doubtful.[1] What causes such rapid digestion of the gut wall as to lead to free perforation into the general peritoneal cavity is unknown.

Microbiology

Ingested organisms (apart from non-pathogenic lactobacilli and candida species) are rapidly destroyed when the gastric pH is less than 4.0, and the peritonitis after perforation of a peptic ulcer is caused by acid-pepsin – not bacterial – digestion of the peritoneum. If, however, operative repair of the perforation is delayed or inefficient, the inevitable paralytic ileus allows lower intestinal aerobic and anaerobic organisms to gain access to the stomach and duodenum, and thence to the peritoneum.

Treatment

Conservative management by gastric aspiration, intravenous fluid replacement and antibiotics was fashionable 30 years ago but has fallen into disrepute, probably because it came to be practised only in poor-risk patients with an inevitably high mortality rate.

Nearly all patients with perforated peptic ulcers should undergo operation after parenteral analgesia, nasogastric intubation, intravenous saline infusion and a peroperative injection of a broad-spectrum antibiotic.

The question remains whether one should simply close the perforation by suture combined with an omental patch (the technique introduced by Roscoe Graham in 1937)[2] or do a definitive curative operation – and if so, which. On the one hand there is a high incidence of recurrent ulcer following simple suture (reaching 65 per cent in men aged 40–64 years)[3] and, on the other hand, suture combined with proximal gastric vagotomy or truncal vagotomy and pyloroplasty are needlessly radical for the majority of patients. This sort of question is difficult to answer by the technique of a random control clinical trial, partly because of the possibility of bias in the selection of patients and surgeons and partly because of ethical considerations of informed consent. As Alexander J. Walt commented in discussion it is difficult to go to a patient and say 'We have to operate on your perforation. We are not sure what operation is best to do. We will draw a card that will tell us. OK?'[4]

A report of a random control trial in 101 selected good-risk patients undergoing simple closure compared with either truncal vagotomy and drainage or proximal gastric vagotomy and suture does not mention consent to randomization.[5] These authors encountered no deaths or major complications in any group, but a significantly increased recurrence rate (23 out of 32) after simple suture compared with other operations (5 out of 66).

A reasonable compromise solution to the question is to do a simple closure for perforated acute ulcers, and a definitive operation for perforated chronic ulcers. This policy will not only reduce the late recurrence rate, but also prevent immediate postoperative complications related to the continued presence of an active ulcer, the most important complication being haemorrhage.

My own preference is pyloroplasty through the perforation in the case of duodenal ulcers and combined with excision of the ulcer in gastric perforations, together with truncal vagotomy. Advanced age and pre-existing cardiac or pulmonary disease do not contra-indicate the policy, as it is the laparotomy itself, and not the nature of the operation, which causes postoperative chest complications.

Infective complications of peptic perforations

Apart from those which may complicate any major laparotomy, infective complications after adequate repair of a peptic perforation are rare. They include subphrenic and other intraperitoneal abscesses and gastric or duodenal fistulae. I will consider these in more detail in chapter 32.

References

1. McNulty CAM, Wise R. Gastric microflora. *Brit Med J* 1985; **291**:367–68.
2. Graham RR. The treatment of perforated duodenal ulcers. *Surg Gynec Obstet* 1937; **64**:235–38.
3. Greco RS, Cahow CE. Alternatives in the management of acute perforated duodenal ulcer. *Am J Surg* 1974; **127**:109–14.
4. Kirkpatrick JR. The role of definitive surgery in the management of perforated duodenal ulcer disease. *Arch Surg* 1976; **110**:1016–20.
5. Boey J, Lee NW, Koo J, Lam PHM, Wong J, Ong GB. Immediate definitive surgery for perforated duodenal ulcers. A prospective controlled trial. *Ann Surg* 1982; **196**:338–44.

19

Cholecystitis and cholangitis

The normal gall bladder is sterile and, even in the presence of symptomatic gall-stones, no bacteria can be isolated from the bile or the gall bladder wall in 70–80 per cent of cases. When, however, the cystic duct is obstructed by a stone, or when stones lodge in the common bile duct, the incidence of contamination by aerobic bacteria of intestinal origin rises steeply. The most frequently encountered bacteria are coliform organisms – *Escherichia coli* and species of *Klebsiella, Proteus* and *Enterobacter.* Enterococci and streptococci of viridans type are common, but anaerobic bacteria are singularly rare considering their huge numbers in the intestine.

Biliary tract pathology

Acute non-calculous cholecystitis

Gangrene and free perforation of the gall bladder in the absence of stones is rare but often lethal. It may occur as a complication of severe operations or trauma, including burns.[1] The aetiology is obscure but may be analagous to the intestinal gangrene which occasionally complicates serious diseases, and which is caused by vascular occlusion in the intestine.

Gall-stones

Gall-stones are common, particularly in obese women who have borne children. Epidemiological data seem to implicate consumption of refined sugar in the diet, whereas alcohol ingestion appears to have a protective effect.[2] Cholesterol and mixed stones are formed by the action of nucleating factors on bile which is saturated with cholesterol, whereas the much more rare pure pigment stones form at an earlier age, and irrespective of sex, in people who suffer from one of the haemolytic diseases. Pixley and his colleagues examined by real-time ultrasonography 632 women recruited from general practice registers and found gall-stones, or previous cholecystectomy, in 25 per cent.[3] They compared these findings with those in 130 vegetarians in whom the incidence was 12 per cent.

Acute calculous cholecystitis

The findings at operation are of an enlarged, oedematous inflamed gall bladder with lightly-adherent omentum. In only approximately 50 per cent of these patients does culture of the bile or gall bladder wall reveal intestinal bacteria, the inflammation in the other patients being presumably caused by transgression of the mucosal barrier by toxic components of bile, notably lysolecithin. The patient presents with pain and tenderness in the right upper quadrant, and an enlarged gall bladder may be palpated. Constitutional disturbances including pyrexia and neutrophil leucocytosis are common, but the patient is seldom seriously ill, systemic sepsis is rare and the natural history of the disease is towards resolution.

Gall-stone jaundice

Although most cases of jaundice in association with gall-stones are caused by impaction of a stone or stones at the lower end of the common bile duct, there are two exceptions. The first is the syndrome described by Mirizzi in Argentina, in which jaundice is caused by the pressure of a distended obstructed gall bladder on the common bile duct. The second exception is the not uncommon coexistence of gall bladder stones with a carcinoma of the head of the pancreas.

Gall-stone jaundice is seldom as deep as that caused by malignant obstruction, and stones in the common bile duct may cause no jaundice at all, although the serum level of alkaline phosphatase is nearly always considerably raised. The bile is usually infected in the presence of common duct stones; this infection may be asymptomatic or it may lead to cholangitis.

Cholangitis

A common cause of bile duct obstruction and infection in India is the presence in the ducts of *Ascaris lumbricoides*.[4] In South-East Asia oriental cholangitis is sometimes idiopathic and is sometimes caused by infestation by the liver fluke (*Clonorchis sinensis*). It is manifested by recurrent attacks of jaundice and sepsis, stones in the hepatic ducts and bile duct strictures.[5] In Western countries, however, acute pyogenic cholangitis is nearly always caused by gall-stone impaction in the lower common bile duct. It is a dangerous condition, often complicated by Gram-negative septicaemia and septic shock.

Chronic calculous cholecystitis

Repeated attacks of acute pyogenic or chemical cholecystitis result in fibrosis and loss of the concentrating and contracting power of the gall bladder. Bacterial infection is not common.

Diagnosis of gall-stones

Ultrasonography

This is the single most valuable investigation. It is quick, cheap, non-invasive and requires no preparation of the patient. It does, however, depend on the presence of a good B-mode or real-time machine and, above all, a skilled operator. It is particularly valuable in detecting dilatation of intra- and extra-hepatic ducts. Cooperberg and Burhenne examined by real-time ultra-sonography 313 patients who were eventually proved to have gall-stones.[6] They found five false negatives and one false positive. In 124 patients examined by both ultrasonography and oral cholecystography, there were five in whom gall-stones were shown by the former method when the cholecystogram was negative. I regard ultrasonography as the first line investigation, and proceed to other investigations only if it is negative.

Oral cholecystography

The patient is instructed to swallow a sachet of iopanoic acid before going to bed and then to have no food or drink before the examination next morning. X-rays of the right upper abdomen will usually reveal the opacified gall bladder in which, in the presence of stones, negative shadows are seen. Gall bladder emptying in response to a meal is often monitored but is of no additional value except for the diagnosis of non-calculous disease. The investigation has limited value in acutely ill patients, particularly in the presence of acute cholecystitis, pancreatitis or jaundice. Non-visualization of the gall bladder is not synonymous with disease.

Intravenous cholecystography

Intravenous infusion over 1 hour of a large dose (16–20g) of iotroxamide opacifies bile ducts and gall bladder unless they are obstructed. Additional information can be obtained by computed tomography of the opacified biliary system, but this adds considerably to the cost of the investigation. It has largely been replaced by other methods which are discussed below.

Cholescintigraphy

One vial of ^{99}technetium-labelled HIDA is injected intravenously in a starved patient suspected of having acute cholecystitis and pictures are taken with a gamma camera after 1 hour. If the gall bladder is not seen, further pictures are taken 2 and 4 hours later. Non-visualization of the gall bladder is diagnostic of cystic duct obstruction, but false positive results are occasionally found. Cholescintigraphy and ultrasonography are the investigations of choice in the diagnosis of acute cholecystitis.

Percutaneous transhepatic cholangiography

In jaundiced patients with clinical and biochemical evidence of cholestasis and a normal clotting screen it is nearly always possible to opacify the biliary tree by introducing a flexible Chiba needle into the liver and injecting contrast medium under image intensifier control during its withdrawal. The investigation carries a small risk of haemorrhage and biliary peritonitis, and the surgeon should be ready to operate on the patient on the same day.

Endoscopic retrograde cholangiography

Expert endoscopists can nearly always cannulate the papilla of Vater and inject contrast medium to opacify the biliary system and pancreatic duct, unless the papilla opens into a duodenal diverticulum. There is a significant risk of pancreatitis and cholangitis, and it is sensible to give the patient a pre-investigation intravenous dose of aprotinin and a cephalosporin.

Treatment of biliary tract obstruction

Acute cholecystitis

It is proper to treat patients under the age of 70 years, who have no other life-threatening disease, with a parenteral cephalosporin, an aminoglycoside or a beta-lactamase-resistant penicillin and to remove the gall bladder on the next convenient operating list. In very old patients, and those with serious medical diseases, operation should be avoided as its mortality is likely to exceed that of patients treated conservatively. If the gall-stones are not radio-opaque, there may be a place for prolonged treatment with chenodeoxycholic or ursodeoxycholic acid.

Prevention of infection after cholecystectomy

All patients should receive a single intravenous dose of an appropriate antibiotic at induction of anaesthesia. The choice of antibiotic depends on which infecting bacteria are suspected. Random control clinical trials have shown that cephalosporins, beta-lactamase-resistant penicillins, aminoglycosides and trimethoprim give better results, in terms of the prevention of postoperative infections, than those of control groups receiving no prophylactic antibiotic.

The influence of operative technique

There is little to choose between a vertical midline or paramedian and a transverse or oblique incision, in terms of either wound healing or chest complications.[7] Unless the common bile duct has been opened there is no advantage in draining the gall bladder bed. In a clinical trial in my unit in 155 consecutive patients randomized to have fine-bore closed suction drainage or no drainage, there were no discernible differences between the groups in terms of infective complications or duration of hospital stay.[8]

In an audit of 224 consecutive patients undergoing cholecystectomy in my unit, 105 had a cholecystectomy alone and in 119 it was accompanied by incidental appendicectomy.[9] In patients receiving prophylactic cephaloridine there was no significant difference in the wound infection rate between the 49 patients without appendicectomy (10.2 per cent) and the 46 patients with appendicectomy (8.7 per cent). When, however, either no prophylactic or an ineffective prophylactic antibiotic was given, the rates were significantly different: 16.1 per cent of 56 patients who did not have the appendix removed, compared with 41.1 per cent of those who did ($P < 0.01$). I have therefore abandoned the practice of incidental appendicectomy during operations which are usually clean.

Treatment of bile duct obstructions

Pre-operative and non-surgical measures

Deep jaundice is more likely to result from malignant obstruction, whereas obstruction by a stone or stones usually results in a lesser degree of jaundice but is more often complicated by cholangitis and septicaemia. The first essential in treatment is therefore to prescribe a parenteral antibiotic which is active against Gram-negative rods (usually *E. coli*). Disturbance of prothrombin synthesis is common, and intramuscular vitamin K should be given. Adequate hydration and urine output are essential – renal impairment is common.

In very old and infirm patients it is desirable to avoid laparotomy; the choice is then between percutaneous catheter drainage of a dilated intrahepatic duct, percutaneous transhepatic placement of an endoprosthesis[10] or endoscopic papillotomy and either evacuation of stones by a stone basket or balloon catheter, or – when the obstruction is by cancer – insertion of an endoprosthesis. All these methods are associated with a high incidence of complications and death, and direct comparisons among them in the form of prospective random control trials are not available. There is, however, an increasing trend towards endoscopic rather than transhepatic interventions, and endoscopic papillotomy is the method of choice for septic jaundiced patients with stones in the common bile duct.

What about the patient with obstructive jaundice who is otherwise fit to withstand a laparotomy? Retrospective audits have suggested that preliminary drainage of the dilated biliary tree allows safer definitive operations, but a prospective random control trial showed a postoperative mortality rate in patients with malignant obstruction of 19 per cent without preliminary transhepatic drainage and 32 per cent after such drainage.[11] Although the figures do not differ significantly in a statistical sense, the trial was abandoned after 70 patients had been entered, and the authors concluded that pre-operative transhepatic drainage confers no advantage.

Surgical treatment of bile duct obstructions

The principles are straightforward: give a pre-operative parenteral antibiotic and a peroperative intravenous infusion of 10 per cent mannitol; remove the cause of the obstruction if you can, or bypass it if you cannot. In the former category are patients with stones in the common bile duct, benign (usually iatrogenic) bile duct strictures, and a few with cholangiocarcinomas and carcinomas of the duodenum. Bypass of the obstruction is necessary in most cases of pancreatic parenchymal carcinoma, which seldom reach the surgeon until they are incurable.

All operations in deeply jaundiced patients are risky, the principal complications being sepsis, renal failure and gastrointestinal bleeding. Seven per cent of operations for benign obstruction and 15 per cent of those for malignant obstruction ended fatally in a series reported recently.[12] Old age, impaired renal function and low levels of serum albumin are associated with even higher death rates.

Supraduodenal or transduodenal choledochotomy for stones

My policy is that stones which can be moved by the surgeon's finger and thumb from the lower end of the common bile duct should be removed by supraduodenal choledochotomy, whereas those which cannot should be approached by an incision in the duodenum. Both methods can cause acute pancreatitis which is often severe and may be complicated by pancreatic and extra-pancreatic abscesses. If, however, supraduodenal choledochotomy fails and is immediately followed by transduodenal exploration, the chances of severe pancreatitis are much increased.

Resection of bile duct strictures

Most benign and some malignant strictures should be resected and the proximal duct should be anastomosed, using the mucosal graft technique and a temporary stent, to a Roux loop of jejunum. Septic complications are common and require antibiotic treatment appropriate to the bacteria cultured from specimens taken during the operation.

Pancreatoduodenectomy for malignant bile duct obstruction

Patients with carcinoma of the head of the pancreas can occasionally, and those with carcinoma of the duodenum or lower common bile duct often, be cured by a Whipple operation. There is no particular advantage either in the short term or the long term in doing a total pancreatectomy. The advantages of avoiding the dangerous anastomosis of pancreatic duct to jejunum and of possibly doing a more radical cancer operation are more theoretical than real and are probably more than balanced by the development of brittle diabetes. Septic complications, with or without anastomotic dehiscences, are common.

Bypass operations for inoperable obstructions

Anastomosis of a distended gall bladder, associated with obstruction by a carcinoma of the head of pancreas, to the stomach or a Roux loop of jejunum will usually relieve jaundice (and, from the patient's point of view more importantly, pruritis) and allow a few months of reasonable health. The incidence of subsequent duodenal obstruction is low and my policy is not to add a gastrojejunostomy. If the gall bladder is contracted, usually as a result of the presence of stones unrelated to the biliary obstruction, it is better to anastomose the common duct to the duodenum or jejunum. Palliation of an inoperable cholangiocarcinoma above the entrance of the cystic duct can usually be achieved by choledochotomy, dilatation of the stricture and insertion of a T-tube.

Conclusions

The biliary tree is sterile but if any part of it is obstructed, invasion by intestinal aerobic bacteria soon occurs. The result is often serious sepsis and death in old or debilitated patients. Antibiotics play a major role in treatment but they must usually be supplemented by removal of the gall bladder or relief of bile duct obstruction.

References

1. Devine RM, Farnell MB, Mucha P. Acute cholecystitis as a complication in surgical patients. *Arch Surg* 1984; **119**:1389–93.
2. Scragg RKR, McMichael AJ, Baghurst PA. Diet, alcohol and relative weight in gall stone disease: a case-control study. *Brit Med J* 1984; **288**:1113–19.
3. Pixley F, Wilson D, McPherson K, Mann J. Effect of vegetarianism on development of gall stones in women. *Brit Med J* 1985; **291**:11–12.
4. Khuroo MS, Zargar SA. Biliary ascariasis: a common cause of biliary and pancreatic disease in an endemic area. *Gastroenterology* 1985; **88**:418–23.
5. Carmona RH, Crass RA, Lim RC Jr, Trunkey DD. Oriental cholangitis. *Am J Surg* 1984; **148**:117–24.
6. Cooperberg PL, Burhenne HJ. Real-time ultrasonography. Diagnostic technique of choice in calculous gall bladder disease. *New Eng J Med* 1980; **302**:1277–79.
7. Greenall MJ, Evans M, Pollock AV. Midline or transverse laparotomy? A random control clinical trial. Part I: Influence on healing. Part II: Influence on postoperative pulmonary complications. *Brit J Surg* 1980; **67**:188–94.
8. Playforth MJ, Sauven P, Evans M, Pollock AV. Suction drainage of the gallbladder bed does not prevent complications after cholecystectomy: a random control clinical trial. *Brit J Surg* 1985; **72**:269–71.
9. Pollock AV, Evans M. Wound sepsis after cholecystectomy: effect of incidental appendicectomy. *Brit Med J* 1977; **i**:20–22.
10. Dooley JS, Dick R, George P, Kirk RM, Hobbs KEF, Sherlock S. Percutaneous transhepatic endoprosthesis for bile duct obstruction: complications and results. *Gastroenterology* 1984; **86**:905–09.
11. McPherson GAD, Benjamin IS, Hodgson HJF, Bowley NB, Allison DJ, Blumgart LH. Pre-operative percutaneous transhepatic biliary drainage: the results of a controlled trial. *Brit J Surg* 1984; **71**:371–75.
12. Keighley MRB, Razay G, Fitzgerald MG. Influence of diabetes on mortality and morbidity following operations for obstructive jaundice. *Ann Roy Coll Surg Eng* 1984; **66**:49–51.

20

Pancreatitis and pancreatic abscess

Acute and chronic pancreatitis are not infections, with the exception of the rare form associated with mumps virus. Bacterial infections in the pancreas and elsewhere are, however, important complications and causes of severe illness.

Aetiology

The two main causes of pancreatitis in Western countries are alcohol and gall stones. The proportion of the one to the other varies from country to country; alcoholic pancreatitis is common in the USA and in France. It is increasing in Scotland and to a lesser extent in England where, however, in my own practice it still accounts for less than 10 per cent of all cases of acute pancreatitis. Alcoholism is by far the commonest cause of chronic pancreatitis, but in some African countries a special form of chronic pancreatitis with pancreatic calculi is found, the aetiology of which is unknown.

Pancreatitis may follow penetrating or blunt abdominal trauma, and a particularly dangerous form occasionally follows operations on the bile ducts or duodenum, including transduodenal sphincterotomy.[1,2]

Rare causes of acute pancreatitis include genetic abnormalities, hyperlipaemia, hyperparathyroidism, aortography, renal transplantation, episodes of severe hypotension and medications, including steroids and frusemide. In Trinidad a common cause of severe pancreatitis is the sting of the scorpion *Tityus trinitatis*: the action of the toxin is still not properly understood.[3]

There remain many cases of acute pancreatitis in which no aetiological agent is discovered. These so-called idiopathic cases appear in all series, their number determined partly by the diligence with which known causes are investigated.

Pathogenesis

Gall-stone migration

Opie published an account of the finding at post-mortem examination of a 3 mm calculus lodged in the ampulla of Vater and blocking both common bile and pancreatic ducts.[4] He described the production of canine pancreatitis by injection of bile into the pancreatic duct, and was the first person to postulate that bile activates the pro-enzymes secreted by the pancreas, resulting in autodigestion of the gland. This is probably true of most pancreatitis associated with gall-stones. These cases are characterized by the multiplicity and small size of the stones, by the wider than average cystic duct and by the existence of a common opening of bile and pancreatic ducts into the duodenum.[5,6] Acosta and Ledesma identified gall-stones ranging from 1 mm to 15 mm in diameter in the faeces of 34 out of 36 patients within 10 days of an attack of acute pancreatitis,[7] and considerably strengthened the view that it is the migration of small stones through the ampulla of Vater which causes pancreatitis.

Pancreatic ischaemia

The activation of pancreatic pro-enzymes, particularly trypsinogen, by bile does not explain the numerous attacks of pancreatitis in patients who do not have gall-stones. Alcohol does not have a selective necrotizing action on the pancreas, and the theory that alcohol relaxes the sphincter of Oddi and allows reflux of duodenal fluid up the pancreatic duct is pure conjecture. Foulis examined microscopic sections of 37 pancreases which showed macroscopic changes of pancreatitis.[8] He found that necrosis and inflammation were concentrated either around the ducts or in the periphery of the lobules, and postulated alternative pathways for the evolution of acute pancreatitis – one by intraduct activation of digestive enzymes, the other by ischaemic micro-infarction associated with shock.

Phospholipase A

The role of phospholipase A in pancreatitis has received much attention.[9] It is a heat-stable enzyme converted from phospholipase by the action of trypsin and calcium. It is found most abundantly in snake venom, and in the pancreas, peritoneum and blood in cases of acute pancreatitis. It converts lecithin to toxic lysolecithin, which has been identified in the pancreas in patients who have died of acute pancreatitis. Lysolecithin kills cells by disintegration of their membranes and allows liberation into the blood stream and peripancreatic tissues of active trypsin, elastase and kallikrein together with the more easily identified amylase and lipase. Neither phospholipase A nor lysolecithin is inhibited by aprotinin and there are no endogenous inhibitors.

Distant manifestations of pancreatitis

Multiple organ failure is a characteristic feature of severe pancreatitis. In common with other causes of shock, it manifests itself in pulmonary failure (arterial hypoxia) followed by renal failure (raised serum concentrations of urea and creatinine), hepatic failure (raised serum levels of hepatic enzymes), gastro-intestinal failure (stress ulceration and bleeding) and cerebral failure (impaired consciousness). These manifestations may be the result of liberation into the general circulation of toxic enzymes in sufficient concentration to cause capillaries to become permeable to plasma proteins. This results in sequestration of fluid and deposition of fibrin in the tissues; the fibrin interferes with tissue oxygenation. An alternative explanation is a hypercoagulable state which may lead to intravascular coagulation and tissue ischaemia.[10]

The role of bacteria

No account of the pathogenesis of acute pancreatitis would be complete without a mention of the role of enterobacteria, particularly in relation to late septic complications. All enterobacteria share a common polysaccharide surface antigen, and techniques have been developed to measure the titre of serum antibodies to this antigen. Kivilaakso and his colleagues studied 38 patients with acute pancreatitis.[11] In 11 mild cases the antibody titre remained low throughout the illness, whereas in those who developed complications it rose during the course of the illness. Bacteria probably play no part in the initiation of an attack, but they may colonize and invade areas of necrotic pancreas. Sepsis is the commonest cause of late deaths in this disease.

Diagnosis

The severity of an attack of acute pancreatitis can vary from so mild that the patient does not need admission to hospital to so fulminating that he is dead before a diagnosis is made. In my personal series of 337 cases of acute pancreatitis there were 75 deaths; in 23 (31 per cent) of these deaths the diagnosis was first made at autopsy. This parallels the experience from Glasgow (Imrie, *personal communication*). In 53 (42 per cent) of 126 deaths from pancreatitis over 11 years the diagnosis was not made during life.

The usual history is of epigastric pain, sometimes felt also in the back, with vomiting. In mild cases the patient is not seriously ill, and tenderness may be confined to the epigastrium or right lower quadrant. In more severe attacks the patient is obviously ill and the abdomen is tender and rigid. The diagnosis is usually made by estimation of the concentration of amylase in the serum, using the starch degradation methods of Somogyi or Phadebas, and accepting a fourfold elevation above the upper limit of normal as diagnostic.

Diagnosis of severity

The mortality rate of a mild attack is nil. The mortality rate of a severe attack is from 20 per cent to 80 per cent. It is clear that considerations of treatment and prognosis require that the clinician be able to grade the severity. The first attempt to do this resulted in the Ranson criteria.[12] Multivariate analysis of 13 features showed that nine variables influenced the outcome of an attack, of which the most potent were age, fluid sequestration and elevation of serum levels of hepatic enzymes together with depression of PaO_2, haematocrit and serum calcium. To these variables must be added diagnostic peritoneal lavage with the finding of discoloured 'toxic broth' in the peritoneal cavity.[13,14]

Treatment

Patients with mild attacks will recover whatever treatment is given, and those patients with the most severe attacks will die despite treatment. The majority of patients, however, will respond to hospital treatment, including parenteral analgesics, oxygen by mask, intravenous fluid replacement and nasogastric intubation.

Glucagon and aprotinin

Glucagon depresses pancreatic exocrine secretions, and aprotinin (Trasylol) neutralizes most proteolytic enzymes. Early uncontrolled or poorly controlled reports were favourable, but a Medical Research Council multicentre random control trial of these drugs against placebo for the treatment of 257 patients with severe pancreatitis disclosed no benefit from either.[15] It is probable that the damage has been done by the time the patient comes under treatment, and aprotinin may have a place in the prophylaxis of pancreatitis in patients undergoing endoscopic or surgical exploration of the common bile duct. This has not been proved.

Other antiprotease therapy

Plasma is a rich source of antiproteolytic enzymes, and clinicians have long held the belief that intravenous infusion of plasma is more effective than other colloids, or crystalloids, in the treatment of acute pancreatitis. Cuschieri and his colleagues published an audit of 239 consecutive patients, 170 of whom were classified as having mild, and 69 as having severe, pancreatitis.[16] In addition to standard treatment they were given two or three units of fresh frozen plasma on the day of admission and one or two units daily for the next 4 days. Five of the patients with mild pancreatitis died (2.9 per cent), and four of the patients with severe pancreatitis died (5.8 per cent).

Antiproteases are found in high concentrations in soya beans and in certain strains of streptomyces. Rats treated with leupeptin, a streptomyces antiprotease, survived experimental acute pancreatitis better than controls treated with aprotinin or saline.[17] No clinical data are available.

Peritoneal dialysis

The theoretical attraction of peritoneal dialysis is that it removes toxic products of pancreatic autolysis before they can be absorbed to cause the failure of distant organs. Early reports were favourable, but a random control clinical trial in 91 patients suffering from severe pancreatitis showed no benefit:[18] 12 of 45 patients in the lavage group died (27 per cent) compared with 13 of 46 patients in the control group (28 per cent). Major complications developed in 17 patients (38 per cent) and 16 patients (35 per cent) respectively. The benefit of dialysis shown in earlier studies may have been the result of the massive fluid infusion which it allows.

Urgent sphincterotomy for gall-stone pancreatitis

If gall-stone pancreatitis is caused by temporary impaction of a stone in the ampulla of Vater and mixing of bile with pancreatic juice, it is tempting to believe that urgent endoscopic[19] or transduodenal[20] sphincterotomy will limit the extent of pancreatic necrosis. Neither method has been subjected to the discipline of a well-conducted random control clinical trial, and most surgeons regard early operations on the common bile duct as dangerous.

Pancreatic resection

When portions of the pancreas are dead they invite bacterial colonization and grave septic complications. The problems of pancreatic resection, however, are first that it is difficult to define necrotic pancreas until late in the course of the disease and, secondly, that the operation has a high mortality rate even when performed by experienced surgeons. Kivilaaskso and his colleagues achieved a mortality rate of 22 per cent after pancreatic resection in patients with severe pancreatitis, compared with 47 per cent in those treated by peritoneal dialysis.[21] Nearly 50 per cent of the survivors in the resection group developed diabetes. Most surgeons are content to advise operation only for local complications and to confine resection to finger debridement of obviously necrotic tissue ('pancreatic necrosectomy').

The place of antibiotics

Antibiotics have not been shown either to prevent or to cure local septic complications. They are best avoided except in brief courses as adjuncts to operations for local complications. In such cases either a beta-lactamase-resistant cephalosporin or an aminoglycoside should be given.

Complications: their detection and treatment

Pulmonary, renal and hepatic function should be monitored by daily laboratory tests; hyperglycaemia, hypoalbuminaemia and hypocalcaemia should be treated. Patients with severe pancreatitis lose weight dramatically, and parenteral feeding is often essential to try and conserve body protein. Despite the most energetic intensive therapy, many patients with multiple system organ failure do not respond to treatment, in which case the implication is that local complications have arisen. Every effort must be made to detect the presence of cysts, necrosis and abscesses and to operate on these patients.

Pseudopancreatic cysts

Ultrasound examination in the acute stages of pancreatitis will often show a collection of fluid behind the stomach. These collections usually resolve but may become encysted, often presenting clinically months after the acute attack, or they may rupture into a neighbouring organ and resolve; occasionally, they rupture into the general peritoneal cavity resulting in pancreatic ascites. Percutaneous drainage under ultrasound guidance is sometimes successful, but may not cure the cyst, and occasionally results in secondary infection. Endoscopic pancreatography should be avoided as it also may cause infection of the cyst. An infected pseudocyst is, however, not nearly as dangerous as a pancreatic abscess. Pseudocysts which are causing severe symptoms or which do not resolve during observation over a period of 2 weeks should be anastomosed to the stomach by a transgastric incision, and necrotic tissue within the cyst should be debrided by the surgeon's finger. Pseudocysts in other parts of the abdomen (usually right or left paracolic gutters) should be drained externally.

Pancreatic necrosis

There is no certain way of diagnosing necrosis in the pancreas or peripancreatic structures until invasion by enteric organisms results in an abscess. Elevation of serum concentration of C-reactive protein is highly suggestive of necrosis but, for localization of the necrosis, computerized tomography with contrast enhancement offers the best chance, and it should be requested at frequent intervals for any patient who remains ill after the first few days. Pancreatic necrosectomy should be performed by an approach through the lesser sac or through the transverse mesocolon. Necrosis of the transverse colon is by no means rare and requires colectomy without anastomosis.

Pancreatic abscesses

These abscesses, caused by invasion of necrotic tissues by intestinal organisms, may complicate any case of severe pancreatitis; they are more often encountered after postoperative pancreatitis than after gall-stone, alcoholic or idiopathic pancreatitis. They differ from most other intra-abdominal abscesses in being frequently multiple or multiloculated, and the successful drainage of a single abscess does not predicate the patient's survival. The mortality rate in most series is high, ranging from 30 per cent to 70 per cent. Warshaw and Jin presented a series of 45 patients whose abscesses were operated on at the Massachusetts General Hospital between 1974 and 1983.[22] In the first 5 years, 10 out of 26 patients died (38 per cent), but in the second 5 years only one out of 19 patients died (5 per cent). They attribute this improvement to more frequent use of computerized tomography and early aggressive operation, preferring the transmesocolic approach, resecting necrotic tissue and leaving several drains in the cavity. Complications were common including recurrent abscesses, pancreatic fistulae and secondary haemorrhage, which was usually lethal.

An alternative approach is offered by Bradley and Fulenwider who advocate a bilateral subcostal incision and make no attempt to close the abdomen after debridement of the abscess.[23] They merely pack the cavity with laparotomy pads which are changed, and further debridement is performed (at first under general anaesthesia), every 2 or 3 days. They treated 21 patients in this way and three patients died. They emphasize that it is the frequent re-laparotomy with debridement which is the essential part of this treatment. This is an attractive concept which is applicable not only to pancreatic abscesses but to other complicated intra-abdominal abscesses.[24]

Any operation for pancreatic abscess should include a gastrostomy and a feeding jejunostomy; the gastrostomy is to save the patient the necessity for prolonged nasogastric intubation, and the jejunostomy is for enteral hyper-alimentation during recovery.

Conclusions

Acute pancreatitis is potentially lethal in elderly people. It is often compli-cated by multiple system organ failure and, occasionally, by the development of peripancreatic cysts or abscesses. Aggressive non-operative treatment in the early stages and vigilance for the development of pancreatic sloughs and abscesses offer patients the best chance of recovery.

References

1. Campbell R, Kennedy T. The management of pancreatic and pancreatico-duodenal injuries. *Brit J Surg* 1980; **67**:845–50.
2. Fitzgibbon TJ, Yellin AE, Maruyama MM, Donovan AJ. Management of the transected pancreas following distal pancreatectomy. *Surg Gynecol Obstet* 1982; **154**:225–31.
3. Bartholomew C, McGeeney KF, Murphy JJ, Fitzgerald O, Sankaran H. Experi-mental studies on the aetiology of acute scorpion pancreatitis. *Brit J Surg* 1976; **63**:807–10.
4. Opie EL. The etiology of acute haemorrhagic pancreatitis. *Bull Johns Hopkins Hosp* 1901; **12**:182–88.
5. McMahon MJ, Playforth MJ, Booth EW. Identification of risk factors for acute pancreatitis from routine radiological investigation of the biliary tract. *Brit J Surg* 1981; **68**:465–67.
6. Armstrong CP, Taylor TV, Jeacock J, Lucas S. The biliary tract in patients with acute gallstone pancreatitis. *Brit J Surg* 1985; **72**:551–55.
7. Acosta JM, Ledesma CL. Gall stone migration as a cause of acute pancreatitis. *New Eng J Med* 1974; **290**:484–87.
8. Foulis AK. Histological evidence of initiating factors in acute necrotizing pancreatitis in man. *J Clin Path* 1980; **33**:1125–31.
9. Nevaleinen TJ. The role of phospholipase A in acute pancreatitis. *Scand J Gastroenterol* 1980; **15**:641–50.
10. Ranson JHC, Lackner H, Berman IR, Schinella R. The relationship of coagulation factors to clinical complications of acute pancreatitis. *Surgery* 1977; **81**:502–11.
11. Kivilaakso E, Valtoren VV, Malkamaki M, Palmu A, Schroder T, Nikki P, Makela PH, Lempinen M. Endotoxaemia and acute pancreatitis: correlation between severity of the disease and the anti-enterobacterial common antigen antibody titre. *Gut* 1984; **25**:1065–70.
12. Ranson JHC, Pasternack BS. Statistical methods for quantifying the severity of clinical acute pancreatitis. *J Surg Res* 1977; **22**:79–91.
13. Mayer AD, McMahon MJ. The diagnostic and prognostic value of peritoneal lavage in patients with acute pancreatitis. *Surg Gynec Obstet* 1985; **160**:507–12.
14. Williamson RCN. Early assessment of severity in acute pancreatitis. *Gut* 1984; **25**:1331–39.
15. Medical Research Council Multicentre Trial. Morbidity of acute pancreatitis: the effect of aprotinin and glucagon. *Gut* 1980; **21**:334–39.

16. Cuschieri A, Wood RAB, Cumming JRG, Meehan SE, Mackie CR. Treatment of acute pancreatitis with fresh frozen plasma. *Brit J Surg* 1983; **70**:710–12.
17. Jones PA, Hermon-Taylor J, Grant DAW. Antiproteinase chemotherapy of acute experimental pancreatitis using the low molecular weight oligopeptide aldehyde leupeptin. *Gut* 1982; **23**:939–43.
18. Mayer AD, McMahon MJ, Corfield AP, Cooper MJ, Williamson RCN, Dickson AP, Shearer MG, Imrie CW. Controlled clinical trial of peritoneal lavage for the treatment of severe acute pancreatitis. *New Eng J Med* 1985; **312**:399–404.
19. Safrary L, Cotton PB. A preliminary report: urgent duodenoscopic sphincterotomy for acute gallstone pancreatitis. *Surgery* 1981; **89**:424–28.
20. Stone HH, Fabian TC, Dunlop WE. Gallstone pancreatitis: biliary tract pathology in relation to time of operation. *Ann Surg* 1981; **194**:305–12.
21. Kivilaakso E, Lempinen M, Makelainen A, Nikki P, Schroder T. Pancreatic resection versus peritoneal lavation for acute fulminant pancreatitis. A randomized prospective study. *Ann Surg* 1984; **199**:426–31.
22. Warshaw AL, Jin G. Improved survival in 45 patients with pancreatic abscess. *Ann Surg* 1985; **202**:408–17.
23. Bradley EL III, Fulenwider JT. Open treatment of pancreatic abscess. *Surg Gynec Obstet* 1984; **159**:509–13.
24. Mughal MM, Bancewicz, J, Irving MH. 'Laparostomy': a technique for the management of intractable intra-abdominal sepsis. *Brit J Surg* 1986; **73**:253–59.

21

Infections of the appendix

The human appendix is a tubular organ, and its narrow lumen (the capacity seldom exceeds 0.5 ml), the thin secretory mucosa, the presence of lymphoid tissue and the relatively thick muscles in the wall all combine to allow obstruction to cause breaches in the mucosal lining and invasion by faecal aerobic and anaerobic organisms.

The vermiform appendix was given that name by Andreas Vesalius in 1543, and physicians have known for centuries that abscesses in the right lower abdomen could occur and could be lethal. In 1769 John Hunter described a gangrenous appendix which he found when he did an autopsy on a Colonel Dalrymple, [1] but strangely enough this great enquirer did not take the matter any further, and 'perityphlitis' remained a medical curiosity until Reginald Heber Fitz of Boston, USA, presented a paper on a new disease which he called appendicitis at the inaugural meeting of the Association of American Physicians in 1886. Although Fitz made a plea for the 'timely and appropriate treatment' of appendicitis, he saw only 72 patients with appendicitis in the next 5 years. [2] In 66 patients the appendix had perforated and the patient presented with an abscess which Fitz drained. In only six patients did he remove the appendix. The mortality rate was 26 per cent. It was not until two decades later that surgeons began routinely removing inflamed appendices without waiting for them to perforate.

Aetiology

The bacteria in the lumen of the appendix are faecal. Numerically, the most prominent are *Bacteroides fragilis*, followed by *Escherichia coli* and other Gram-negative rods. Enterococci and other aerobic and anaerobic streptococci are commonly isolated, as is *Clostridium perfringens*. When the mucosa of the appendix is breached the resultant inflammation of the wall of the organ is caused by synergistic growth of aerobic and anaerobic bacteria. [3] I know of no adequate explanation for the fact that inflammation of the appendix is always transmural, whereas inflammation in the rest of the colon is usually confined to the mucosa and submucosa.

Geographical distribution

In Europe, North America and Australia appendicitis is the most frequently encountered of all the intra-abdominal infections. It is rare in countries with a lower standard of living and a higher ratio of rural to city dwellers. Friedlander and Gelfand reported that in 1975 in Harare, Zimbabwe, 604 white and 95 black people were admitted to hospital with appendicitis. [4] Only 22 of the blacks were from rural communities.

Genetic and familial factors

It is not uncommon for siblings of a child whose appendix has been removed to present with appendicitis. This may, however, merely be due to a heightened awareness of the disease on the part of the parents. There is no evidence that races differ in their inherent susceptibility to appendicitis; black people resident in North America, and immigrants from countries with a low incidence of the disease, all suffer the disease as frequently as whites.

Dietary factors

The only acceptable hypothesis to explain the increased incidence of the disease in the last 100 years, and the geographical distribution, is that there is something in the twentieth century Western diet which predisposes to appendicitis. Sixty years ago Short found that well-fed children in private boarding schools had a higher incidence of appendicitis than those in orphanages, [5] and Burkitt put forward cogent epidemiological arguments for the role of refined carbohydrates and the removal of fibre from foods in the aetiology of the disease.[5]

Pathology

Luminal obstruction by a faecolith or by swelling of the lymphoid tissue in the wall of the appendix is probably the first event. This is the only reasonable explanation for the colicky abdominal pain which heralds attacks of appendicitis, and for the fact that proximal inflammation without distal involvement is never seen, although inflammation confined to the tip of the appendix is quite common.

At one time a distinction was made between catarrhal appendicitis, which tended to recover, and obstructive appendicitis, which tended to progress to gangrene and perforation. This distinction is seldom made nowadays, although it is still recognized that many attacks of appendicitis go on to resolution. Arnbjornson and Bengmark, however, have revived the theory that infection may cause obstruction rather that vice versa. [6] They measured the pressure in the appendix during operation by needle and water manometer. They found that the pressure was zero in five normal organs and in 19 out of 21 acutely inflamed appendices, but over 20 cm H_2O in gangrenous organs. These observations need to be verified.

Clinical features

Non-perforated appendicitis

The classical presentation of colicky diffuse abdominal pain with nausea and anorexia, going on to localization of the pain in the right lower quadrant, is seen in about 50 per cent of all cases. A complaint of headache is so rare that its presence practically excludes appendicitis. Atypical presentations are common and, in the words of Berry and Malt, 'Just as surgeons . . . did a century ago, we now diagnose acute appendicitis by clinical instinct'. [2] There are no absolute rules for the diagnosis of appendicitis, and surgeons must accept that they are going to remove some normal appendices rather than leave a patient in whom they are doubtful of the diagnosis to suffer perforation of the organ.

Increasing diagnostic accuracy is accompanied by an increased rate of perforation[2] and, in young people particularly, surgeons should be prepared to find that 30 per cent of the appendices removed are normal. In these cases the true pathology ranges from so-called non-specific abdominal pain, which is usually accompanied by psychological changes, through mesenteric adenitis and enteritis to any of the numerous causes of right-sided abdominal peritoneal irritation. These include sealed leaks from duodenal ulcers, mild acute pancreatitis, acute cholecystitis, Meckel's or solitary caecal diverticulitis, acute Crohn's or *Yersinia* ileo-colitis and pelvic inflammatory disease. The higher rate of removal of normal appendices in young women reflects the diagnostic confusion caused by tubovarian conditions.

In auditing a recent personal consecutive series of 313 appendicectomies for acute abdominal pain I found that 31 per cent of the appendices were histologically normal. When I analysed the age and sex distribution in this series, it turned out that 46 per cent of 147 appendices in women under the age of 50 years were normal, compared with 17 per cent of 101 appendices in young men. Over the age of 50 years this difference was less marked, normal appendices being removed from 23 per cent of 35 older women and 13 per cent of 30 older men; this difference is not significant. The incidence of appendicular perforation also varied by age and sex. Young women had the lowest incidence (14 per cent), followed by young men (25 per cent). Older women (43 per cent) and older men (53 per cent) were significantly more likely to have perforated appendices removed.

Perforated appendicitis

Patients with perforated appendicitis present in one of three ways. If the gangrenous organ has been effectively isolated by fibrinous adhesions to surrounding omentum and intestine, the patient presents with a fixed mass in the right lower quadrant unaccompanied by severe constitutional signs of infection. Secondly, less absolute encapsulation by surrounding tissues results in local peritonitis with pus. Finally, reflecting either a primary failure of the host to localize the perforation or a secondary failure of the containing barrier – sometimes caused by ill-advised prescription of aperients or enemas – the patient may present with general peritonitis and toxaemia. It is mainly in the latter group that the lethal results of appendicitis are found; about 100 people die of appendicitis every year in England and Wales. [7]

Treatment

Only if the bedside examination shows a fixed mass in the right lower quadrant should appendicectomy be avoided. These patients do well with conservative treatment, and the appendix should be removed a month or so later. In all other cases it is necessary to remove the appendix, preferably by a transverse muscle-splitting incision at about umbilical level. It does not seem to matter whether the stump is cauterized, inverted or left alone.

Antibiotics

Once the acutely inflamed appendix has been removed, the peritoneum is quite capable of looking after itself. The purpose of antibiotic prophylaxis is to minimize the effects of parietal contamination by faecal organisms. Such contamination is common, even if the appendix is normal. It is more frequent during removal of a gangrenous appendix, and it always complicates removal of a perforated appendix. Every patient undergoing appendicectomy should therefore be given a pre-operative antibiotic by intramuscular or intravenous injection or, in the case of metronidazole, by suppository. The choice of antibiotic should take into account the synergism between coliform organisms and *B. fragilis*, but random control clinical trials have not shown any advantage of either metronidazole alone or one of the beta-lactamase-resistant antibiotics alone. My preference, particularly when clinical examination suggests that the appendix has perforated, is to give both metronidazole and a third-generation cephalosporin such as latamoxef or the combination of amoxycillin with clavulanic acid (Augmentin). A single preoperative dose is all that is needed except when the appendix has perforated, when two more doses should be given.

Peritoneal lavage or dialysis

The idea of washing away pus and bacteria from the peritoneal cavity and abdominal wall is a survival of the Halsted tradition and, whereas the mechanical removal of particulate contamination is required during operations for faecal peritonitis from colonic perforations, there is no evidence that lavage with or without an antibiotic added to the fluid is of any value in the treatment of perforated appendicitis. [8]

Intraperitoneal drainage

Provided the appendix has been removed it is not necessary, and may be disadvantageous, to leave a drain or drains in the peritoneal cavity. [9]

Skin closure

When pus is encountered during the removal of an appendix by a transverse muscle-splitting incision, it is wise to leave the skin unsutured. If the wound is absolutely clean on the fifth day, the edges may be drawn together with adhesive tapes, but even if healing is allowed to proceed by granulation, it is nearly always complete within 1 month and leaves a linear scar. [10]

Complications

The most common complication is wound infection, the rate being proportional to the degree of peroperative parietal contamination. Serious intra-abdominal sepsis is rare, and the only common abscess sites are in the appendix fossa and the pelvis. These abscesses often discharge spontaneously either through the wound or through the rectum. Intestinal obstruction occasionally follows the ileus of peritonitis and may require surgical intervention.

Conclusions

Acute appendicitis is one of the commonest diseases in countries with a 'Western' refined diet. An attack may resolve or go on to gangrene or perforation. Treatment by appendicectomy after a single dose of an antibiotic – or, in seriously ill patients, of two antibiotics to combat both aerobic and anaerobic bacterial invasion – is usually followed by an uncomplicated recovery.

References

1. Williams GR. A history of appendicitis with anecdotes illustrating its importance. *Ann Surg* 1983; **187**:495–506.
2. Berry J Jr, Malt RA. Appendicitis near its centenary. *Ann Surg* 1984; **200**:567–575.
3. Altemeier WA. The pathogenicity of the bacteria of appendicitis peritonitis. An experimental study. *Surgery* 1942; **11**:374–384.
4. Friedlander ML, Gelfand M. Acute appendicitis, an urban disease in Africans. *Tropical Doctor* 1981; **11**:22–23.
5. Burkitt DP. The aetiology of appendicitis. *Brit J Surg* 1971; **58**:697–699.
6. Arnbjörnson E, Bengmark S. Role of obstruction in the pathogenesis of acute appendicitis. *Am J Surg* 1984; **147**:390–392.
7. Charlton JRH, Prochazka A, Lakhani A. Death from appendicitis outside hospital. *Lancet* 1984; **2**:399.
8. Sauven P, Playforth MJ, Smith GMR, Evans M, Pollock AV. Single dose antibiotic prophylaxis of abdominal surgical wound infection: a trial of preoperative latamoxef against peroperative tetracycline lavage. *J Roy Soc Med* 1986; **79**:137–141.
9. Greenall MJ, Evans M, Pollock AV. Should you drain a perforated appendix? *Brit J Surg* 1978; **65**:880–882.
10. Brennan SS, Smith GMR, Evans M, Pollock AV. The management of the perforated appendix: a controlled clinical trial. *Brit J Surg* 1982, **69**:510–512.

22

Inflammatory bowel diseases

Although it appears to be fragile, the mucosa of the small and large intestine has remarkable powers of preventing invasion by any of the miriad of intestinal bacteria. The barrier can, however, be breached not only by specific microorganisms or their toxins, but also by several diseases which are not primarily bacterial in origin. These include ischaemic enterocolitis, Crohn's enterocolitis, ulcerative colitis, colonic diverticular disease and irradiation damage to the bowel.

Specific enterocolitides

With few exceptions these occur when ignorance and poverty are allied with overcrowding. Enteropathic viruses, bacteria, protozoa and helminths are transmitted by faecal contamination of food and water, and are important causes of death, particularly in infants in tropical countries. From the surgical point of view they are important for several reasons: first, they must be considered in the differential diagnosis of inflammatory and malignant diseases which require surgical intervention. Secondly, they may be complicated by perforation and metastatic abscesses. Thirdly, the responsible microorganisms may contaminate endoscopes and cause cross infection.[1] For detailed discussion of the non-surgical aspects of specific enterocolitides I refer the reader to standard works[2] and propose restricting myself to some of the conditions which are of direct concern to surgeons.

Typhoid perforation

In a report from Benares, more than half of all gastro-intestinal perforations admitted to a surgical unit were the result of typhoid, and the mortality rate was 47 per cent.[3] Early laparotomy with exteriorization of the site of perforation is essential, together with antibiotic treatment, usually by chloramphenicol.

Dysentery

Both bacterial (Shigella) and amoebic dysentery may be mistaken for ulcerative colitis, and both may, occasionally, be complicated by toxic megacolon and perforation. Chronic infection with *Entamoeba histolytica* in the caecum may result in an amoeboma which must be distinguished from a carcinoma and must be treated with metronidazole and not by resection, which carries a high mortality rate. Amoebic liver abscesses are common in regions of endemic amoebiasis, and they require aspiration and 10 days of oral metronidazole 1 g twice daily.

Pseudomembranous (antibiotic-associated) colitis

Thirty years ago, when antibiotics were first used in large quantities, this was known as staphylococcal enterocolitis, and it was not until 1977 that Bartlett and his colleagues recognized that the disease is caused by *Clostridium difficile* which produces a cytopathic exotoxin, the effects of which are neutralized by *Clostridium sordelii* antitoxin.[4] The course of the disease, which may complicate treatment by any antibiotic (clindamycin has the worst reputation), varies from mild to fulminating. Diarrhoea is the main presenting symptom, and the diagnosis is made by sigmoidoscopy which shows patchy plaques of pseudomembrane on the rectal mucosa. Histologically, the changes of acute inflammation are seen. *C. difficile* can be cultured, but the most sensitive and specific test is the detection of the cytopathic effect of its exotoxin on tissue cultures of fibroblasts.

Severe cases of antibiotic-associated colitis should be treated by oral vancomycin 125 mg four times daily for 14 days, supplemented by oral cholestyramine 4 g four times daily. Relapses are common and require further treatment. Metronidazole and bacitracin have been reported to be effective as alternatives to vancomycin.

Ileocolic tuberculosis

This is an important cause of ill health and of intestinal obstruction, perforation and fistula formation in developing countries. Although all tuberculous disease is rare in Western countries, it must be considered in immigrants particularly in the differential diagnosis of Crohn's disease; the pathological lesions are similar, and even the histological picture is not entirely specific – when caseation is present the lesion is certainly tuberculous, but some tuberculomas have very little or no caseation. Clinically, the presence of ascites in association with an inflammatory mass in the ileum or colon is highly suggestive of tuberculosis, and laparoscopic biopsy may prove conclusive. In Western countries, however, the diagnosis is frequently not made until laparotomy with or without excision of the involved bowel. Antituberculous chemotherapy should then be instituted. To prescribe corticosteroids in the mistaken belief that the disease is Crohn's disease is to court disaster.

Yersinia infections

The finding of acute terminal ileitis at operation for presumed appendicitis should raise the suspicion of infection with *Yersinia enterocolitica* or the rarer infection with *Yersinia pseudotuberculosis*. The lesion cannot be distinguished macroscopically from acute Crohn's disease and, as neither microbiological nor histological data are available in most cases, it is possible that many cases which are labelled acute Crohn's ileitis are in fact the result of *Yersinia* infection. Both conditions are self-limiting and require no specific treatment.

Campylobacter infection

Many normal appendices are removed from young people who may be suffering from acute gastroenteritis as a result of infection with *Campylobacter*. The organism can be grown from faeces on specific media, and the disease is normally self-limiting. Severe cases may require erythromycin treatment.

Infantile necrotizing enterocolitis

In neonatal intensive care units in which an aggressive policy of rescue of premature babies is followed, sporadic and, occasionally, epidemic cases of necrotizing enterocolitis occur.[5] The case fatality rate varies from 20 per cent to 40 per cent; death is caused by septicaemia, intestinal obstruction or perforation. The fundamental cause is a failure of the intestinal, and sometimes the right colonic, wall to resist the invasion of bacteria from the lumen. The nature of the defect remains obscure, as does the nature of the causative bacteria. It was thought that clostridia, either *C. perfringens* or *C. difficile* were responsible, but these organisms are as frequently isolated from the faeces of normal neonates as from victims of necrotizing enterocolitis. There is some evidence that *Klebsiella* species may be responsible, and that cross infection within an intensive care unit can occur.

Surgically significant worm infestations

In hot countries *Ascaris lumbricoides* is a common cause of childhood intestinal obstruction.[6] The worms may also cause obstructive jaundice and cholangitis by migrating into the common bile duct. Apart from these syndromes, and the rare pseudotumours caused by penetration of the intestine by the larvae of several other species of round worm, the main surgical importance of infestations is that a patient with a heavy worm burden is likely to be debilitated and to stand major operations poorly.

Ischaemic enterocolitis

The efficient functioning of the intestinal mucosal barrier against infection depends on a generous supply of oxygenated blood. The syndromes of ischaemic enterocolitis encompass many clinical manifestations. On the one hand embolic or thrombotic occlusion of the superior mesenteric artery may cause death of most of the small – and the right half of the large – intestine; patchy necrosis of the small bowel is a feature of enteritis necroticans, the so-called pig bel of Papua New Guinea; non-occlusive intestinal gangrene is sometimes seen *post mortem* in patients who have died unexpectedly after apparent recovery from serious diseases or abdominal operations; finally, there is the syndrome of ischaemic colitis which may recover completely or heal with stricturing, or may be followed by perforation, peritonitis or abscess.

Intestinal infarction

Acute occlusion of the superior mesenteric artery by an embolus (which usually lodges beyond tne origin of the middle colic artery), or by atheromatous thrombosis (usually at the origin of the superior mesenteric artery), results in death of a large part of the intestine. A far less common cause of intestinal infarction is diffuse venous thrombosis. More distal arterial occlusions cause more limited areas of intestinal gangrene.

These patients can be rescued only by early operation, before the onset of bacterial peritonitis, and the diagnosis must always be suspected in a patient whose abdominal pain is excessive in relation to the physical signs. Such a patient should be given 10 000 units of heparin by intravenous injection when first seen, together with intravenous gentamicin 120 mg and metronidazole 500 mg.

Two diagnostic tests are useful – first, the finding of an excess of polymorphonuclear leucocytes in a stained film of the sediment of effluent from a diagnostic peritoneal lavage means that there is an inflammatory process within the peritoneal cavity, and it is an indication for immediate laparotomy. The second test, specific for mesenteric occlusion, is a selective angiogram which will show the site and often the nature of the occlusion. If, however, its performance would delay laparotomy it is safer to forgo it: superior mesenteric occlusion is one of the few true surgical emergencies.

Intestine which is obviously gangrenous must be resected, and every effort must be made to restore the blood supply to ischaemic, but potentially viable, gut. When the occlusion is embolic this is relatively easy – the middle colic artery is traced to its origin, the superior mesenteric artery incised and the embolus extracted by an embolectomy catheter. If the occlusion is the result of atheromatous thrombosis, an aorto-mesenteric reversed saphenous vein graft is required. In any patient in which gangrenous intestine has been resected, it is safer to exteriorize both ends of the bowel and not perform a primary anastomosis. If this is done, there is no need to re-open the abdomen after 24 hours to confirm viability of the remaining gut.

Ischaemic colitis

Ischaemic colitis is rarely caused by occlusion of the inferior mesenteric artery, which may complicate aortic occlusive disease and aneurysm, and is usually asymptomatic. In most cases, no major arterial occlusion is found, and the cause appears to be a failure of the peripheral arterial supply to the left colon, particularly just distal to the splenic flexure.

Ischaemic colitis causes abdominal pain and bloody diarrhoea. When the ischaemia is limited to the mucosa there are no signs of peritonitis. When it is transmural, however, the signs indicate the presence of local peritonitis, but this seldom ends in perforation with general purulent peritonitis or abscess. Patchy mucosal infarction and oedema can be recognized on plain abdominal X-rays – the sign known as 'thumb-printing'. Rigid sigmoidoscopy rarely shows any change in the lower 25 cm of colon, but flexible sigmoidoscopy will allow visualization of sloughs and ulcers in the descending colon. Barium enema X-rays are mainly of value in excluding cancer as the cause of the symptoms.

The treatment of ischaemic colitis is primarily medical, and complete recovery is the rule, although symptomatic or asymptomatic strictures of the upper descending colon may need surgical treatment later. Medical treatment includes rest, attention to fluid requirements and administration of antibiotics active against intestinal aerobic and anaerobic bacteria. Anticoagulant treatment does not appear to shorten the course of the disease. Surgical intervention may be required for the rare cases of frank colonic perforation and for the resection of a late stricture. In the presence of pus, the affected bowel should be resected and the ends exteriorized, anastomosis being delayed until sepsis has resolved.

Crohn's disease and ulcerative colitis

The term 'inflammatory bowel disease' is commonly used to refer to these conditions. Although it is usually possible to distinguish between them, there are a few cases of colitis in which even examination of the whole of a resected specimen results in an indeterminate diagnosis. The World Organization of Gastroenterology Research Committee analyzed the data from 1696 patients in 16 countries and produced a scoring system (Table 22.1) which allows an accuracy of over 90 per cent in separating the two conditions.[7] A high positive score favours Crohn's disease and a high negative score favours ulcerative colitis.

Aetiology

The aetiology of these diseases is unknown; there is no animal model of either disease, and conjectures are based largely on epidemiological studies.[8] Genetic factors are suggested by the fact that the diseases are commoner in white people than in black people, and in Ashkenazi Jews than in Gentiles. Jews in Israel, however, do not have a higher incidence of these diseases than is found elsewhere in the Western world, and the apparent genetic factors may reflect environmental differences. Dietary factors have received considerable attention, but the exact nature of the predisposing diet has not been defined. Kirsner and Shorter reviewed the subject extensively, and concluded that the 'best guess' at present is that the diseases are caused by an interaction between external agents, host responses and immunological influences.[9] Ulcerative colitis (but not Crohn's disease) appears to be one of the few diseases which is less common in cigarette smokers, but the association may be with giving up smoking rather than with not smoking.[10,11] Bacterial invasion is important in the pathogenesis of the complications of both diseases.

Table 22.1 Score system for the differential diagnosis of Crohn's disease and ulcerative colitis

Age			Tenderness	
< 19 years	+ 1		right lower quadrant	+ 10
50–59 years	− 1		upper half	− 2
> 70 years	− 2		left half	− 3
			central	+ 6
Duration			nil	− 1
1–3 months	− 2			
3–6 months	− 1		Abdominal findings	
			distension	+ 2
Family history			mass	+ 10
ulcerative colitis	− 2			
Crohn's disease	+ 4		Radiology	
appendicitis	+ 3		normal	− 3
anal fissure	+ 7		continuous	− 1
fistula	+ 4		segmental	+ 11
nil	− 1		site	
			jejunum	+ 7
Site of pain			ileum	+ 31
right lower quadrant	+ 10		right colon	+ 1
left lower quadrant	− 1		left colon	− 1
right half	+ 2		rectum	− 3
left half	− 6		findings	
central	+ 2		stenosis	+ 4
nil	− 1		ulcers	− 1
			dilatation	+ 4
Type of pain			fistula	+ 6
severe	+ 2		skip lesions	+ 8
steady	+ 2			
			Endoscopy	
Bowels			normal	+ 12
normal	+ 1		ulcers	− 1
diarrhoea			stenosis	+ 2
× 1 per day	+ 3		bleeding	− 4
× > 10 per day	− 2		diffuse	− 2
			patchy	+ 16
Blood				
nil	+ 6		Biopsy	
slight	− 2		normal	+ 5
considerable	− 5		ulcers	− 3
			giant cells	+ 20
Mucus			granulomas	+ 27
nil	+ 3		mucosal inflammation	− 1
slight	− 1		transmural inflammation	+ 16
considerable	− 2			
			Laboratory tests	
Complications			haemoglobin < 10 g/dl	− 1
perianal	+ 7		white cell count > 20 × 10^9/litre	+ 1
fistula	+ 8		albumin > 50 g/litre	− 1
systemic	+ 1		platelets < 150 × 10^9/litre	− 6
			> 400 × 10^9/litre	+ 1
Nutrition				
emaciated	+ 2			

This table is adapted from the *British Medical Journal* 1982; **284**:91–96 by permission of the publishers.

Complications

Both diseases can cause chronic ill health. Anaemia, weight loss, hypo-proteinaemia and, in children, retardation of growth are constant accompaniments of severe active disease. On the other hand, ulcerative colitis confined to the rectum, and inactive primary or recurrent Crohn's disease, are compatible with a normal healthy life. The local complications are to some extent shared by the two diseases, but there are some which reflect both the proclivity of Crohn's disease to affect the small bowel, and its greater tendency towards transmural inflammation and fibrosis.

Bleeding

Massive bleeding may complicate either disease, and it is usually an indication for excisional surgery.

Perforation

Crohn's disease has a much greater tendency than ulcerative colitis to cause local perforation of the gut, resulting in abscess formation or internal or external fistulae. Both diseases can be complicated by toxic dilatation of the colon which, if unrelieved, can result in multiple perforations, general peritonitis and death. Seriously ill patients should have daily plain abdominal X-rays to allow an early diagnosis of toxic megacolon.

Stricture

Strictures represent the fibrotic reaction to transmural Crohn's disease; they are a constant feature in the small bowel and in the rare cases of oesophageal and duodenal disease. A colonic stricture in a patient with chronic ulcerative colitis should raise the suspicion of carcinoma.

Carcinoma

Long-standing inflammatory bowel disease predisposes to the development of carcinoma of the colon or, less often, the small intestine. The incidence is low overall, and the complication arises only when the whole colon is involved and the disease has been present for more than 10 years. It is usually preceded by severe dysplasia or villous adenomatous changes in rectal or colonic biopsies. The 5-year survival does not differ from that of cancer without preceding inflammatory bowel disease – about one third of the patients operated on will be alive after 5 years.[12]

Anal lesions

Painful anal fissures, oedematous skin tags and perianal abscesses and fistulae may be the presenting feature in Crohn's disease; they are seldom seen in ulcerative colitis.

Distant complications

Extra-intestinal manifestations of both diseases are common and involve the skin (erythema nodosum and pyoderma gangrenosum), the eyes (uveitis), the joints (enteropathic arthritis and sacro-iliitis), the kidneys (stones) and the liver (numerous lesions varying from non-specific derangement of liver function tests, to cirrhosis and bile duct carcinoma).

Diagnosis

The diagnosis is made clinically, histologically (rectal or colonic biopsy) and radiologically (Table 22.1). Clinical examination includes sigmoidoscopy, which may be normal in Crohn's disease but usually shows an opaque, granular, friable mucosa in ulcerative colitis. Histologically, the finding of non-caseating granulomas is specific for Crohn's disease, but they are found in only about 25 per cent of all cases. Apart from this, the differential diagnosis of the two conditions on rectal biopsies can be difficult, but goblet cell preservation and submucosal inflammatory cell infiltrates favour Crohn's disease, whereas goblet cell depletion and crypt abscesses favour ulcerative colitis.

   Radiological studies by double-contrast barium enema and barium meal follow-through may be completely normal in ulcerative colitis confined to the rectum, but will show loss of haustral pattern, mucosal ulcers and intervening islands of hypertrophied mucosa in diffuse ulcerative colitis. Crohn's disease of the colon typically spares lengths of gut, normal-looking bowel separating regions of narrowing with fissuring and, sometimes, deeper ulcers or even fistulae. In ileal Crohn's disease the typical findings are long strictures, cobblestone mucosa and deep fissures.

Medical treatment

Both diseases should be treated medically, surgical intervention being reserved for the complications. Antibiotics play no part except as adjuncts to surgical operations.

Ulcerative colitis

This is a disease of remissions and exacerbations. The aims of medical management are, therefore, twofold: to treat exacerbations and to maintain remissions. Mild and distal colitis can be treated in out-patients with daily enemas of prednisolone metasulphobenzoate (Predenema) or hydrocortisone acetate foam in aerosol (Colifoam). This should be continued for 2 weeks and be supplemented by oral sulphasalazine 2 g daily, which should be continued indefinitely to postpone recurrences. Patients with more severe attacks (judged by the severity of symptoms, or the presence of pyrexia, raised erythrocyte sedimentation rate and reduced level of serum albumin) should be admitted to hospital for intravenous fluid and electrolyte replacement, intravenous prednisolone 60 mg daily, and oral sulphasalazine 2 g daily.

Failure to respond to this treatment after 5 days is an indication for urgent colectomy.

The problem of intolerance to sulphasalazine

It is the sulphapyridine component of the molecule which is responsible for most of the toxic effects of sulphasalazine, the therapeutically active component being 5-aminosalicylic acid (5ASA) which is insoluble, unstable and does not reach the colon when given by mouth. In patients intolerant of sulphasalazine there are several less toxic alternatives. Azodisalicylate comprises two molecules of 5ASA united by a diazo bond. It is effective when given by mouth.[13] Two preparations of 5ASA (Pentasa, Asacol) are formulated in such a way that they escape degradation and absorption in the upper gastro-intestinal tract. Finally, 4-aminosalicylic acid is water-soluble, can be given in enema form, and is probably as effective as 5ASA.[14]

Crohn's disease

Inactive Crohn's disease requires no treatment. The mainstays of the medical treatment of active disease are oral prednisolone, sulphasalazine and azathioprine, and evidence is accumulating that cyclosporin may be effective. Widespread small intestinal disease sometimes responds to an elemental diet and may even require total parenteral nutrition.

Surgical treatment

It is important to remember two fundamental differences between ulcerative colitis and Crohn's disease. First, ulcerative colitis can be permanently cured by removal of the whole of the mucosa of the colon and rectum, whereas Crohn's disease is diffuse from the start and cannot be cured – merely held in check. Secondly, the inflammation in Crohn's disease is transmural, and the disease is not influenced by mucosectomy.

Patients with ulcerative colitis who fail to respond to medical treatment, or who suffer frequent debilitating relapses, require total colectomy with a terminal eversion ileostomy. The rectum should not be removed at the primary operation because it is possible in many cases to re-establish intestinal continuity by either an ileorectal or an ileo-anal anastomosis, the latter after mucosal proctectomy with an ileal pouch.[15]

Unresponsive or complicated Crohn's disease of the colon should usually be treated by proctocolectomy. Delayed healing of the perineal wound is to be expected. Crohn's disease of the small intestine, however, requires minimal resection or even, when the indication is stricturing, no resection but strictureplasty.[16] It is not necessary to remove all microscopically detected disease; extensive resections bring the additional problems of intestinal insufficiency.

Diverticular disease of the colon

Infection plays no part in the pathogenesis of diverticular disease unless it is complicated by perforation or chronic inflammation leading to stricturing.

Perforation, which is much more common in the sigmoid than elsewhere in the colon, may result in one of three clinical syndromes – fistula (commonly into the bladder), abscess or general peritonitis. All three syndromes require surgical treatment.

For fistulae, sigmoid resection with anastomosis after mechanical and anti-bacterial bowel preparation is safe. Abscesses should be treated initially by drainage but, if a colocutaneous fistula arises after drainage, the diseased bowel must be resected. Again, primary anastomosis is safe. In the presence of general peritonitis, resection without anastomosis (usually a Hartmann type of operation) is to be preferred because of the danger of anastomotic breakdown.[17]

Irradiation damage to the bowel

Pelvic radiotherapy, mainly for carcinoma of the cervix but also of the bladder, prostate or rectum, can result in acute or delayed ileitis and proctocolitis. In the early stages the condition is associated with hyperaemia and inflammatory infiltration throughout the bowel wall, whereas later in its course the lesions are characterized by arteriolar occlusions, ischaemic fibrosis, fistulae and, curiously enough, sometimes massive haemorrhage.[18]

Resection is usually required for these manifestations, but anastomoses are liable to fail. Failure can be avoided either by not performing an anastomosis or by making sure that at least one end of the resected bowel is outside the irradiated area.[19] Rectovaginal fistula, a common lesion, often implies residual or recurrent cancer as well as irradiation damage, and it is best treated by abdomino-perineal excision of the rectum and vagina or, if this is unacceptable,by colo-anal sleeve anastomosis.

References

1. O'Connor HJO, Axon ATR. Gastro-intestinal endoscopy: infection and disin-fection. *Gut* 1983; **24**:1067–77.
2. Bouchier IAD, Allan RN, Hodgson HJF, Keighley MRB (eds). *Textbook of Gastroenterology*. Baillière Tindall, London, 1984, pp. 1023–1149.
3. Khanna AK, Misra MK. Typhoid perforation of the gut. *Postgrad Med J* 1984; **60**:523–25.
4. Bartlett JG, Anderdonk AB, Cisneros AB, Kasper DL. Clindamycin-associated colitis due to toxin-producing species of clostridium in hamsters. *J Infect Dis* 1977; **136**:701–705.
5. de Louvois J. Necrotising enterocolitis. *J Hosp Infect* 1986; **7**:4–12.
6. Ihekwaba FN. Intestinal ascariasis and the acute abdomen in the tropics. *J Roy Coll Surg Edin* 1980; **25**:452–56.
7. Clamp SE, Myren J, Bouchier IAD, Watkinson G, de Dombal FT. Diagnosis of inflammatory bowel disease: an international multicentre scoring system. *Br Med J* 1982; **284**:91–95.
8. Mayberry JF, Rhodes J. Epidemiological aspects of Crohn's disease: a review of the literature. *Gut* 1984; **25**:886–99.
9. Kirsner JB, Shorter RG. Recent developments in 'non-specific' inflammatory bowel disease. *New Eng J Med* 1982; **306**:837–48.
10. Logan RFA, Edmond M, Somerville KW, Langman MJS. Smoking and ulcera-tive colitis. *Br Med J* 1984; **288**:751–53.

11. Kennedy HG. Smoking and ulcerative colitis. *Br Med J* 1984; **288**:1307.
12. Gyde SN, Prior P, Thompson H, Waterhouse JAH, Allan RN. Survival of patients with colorectal cancer complicating ulcerative colitis. *Gut* 1984; **25**:228–31.
13. Lauritsen K, Hansen J, Ryde M, Rask-Madsen J. Colonic azodisalicylate metabolism determined by *in vivo* dialysis in healthy volunteers and patients with ulcerative colitis. *Gastroenterol* 1984; **86**:1496–1500.
14. Selby WS, Bennett MK, Jewell DP. Topical treatment of distal ulcerative colitis with 4-amino-salicyclic acid enemas. *Digestion* 1984; **29**:231–34.
15. Nicholls J, Pescatori M, Motson RW, Pezim ME. Restorative proctocolectomy with a three loop ileal reservoir for ulcerative colitis and familial adenomatous polyposis. *Ann Surg* 1984; **199**:383–88.
16. Lee ECG. Aim of surgical treatment of Crohn's disease. *Gut* 1984; **25**:217–22.
17. Krukowski ZH, Matheson NA. Emergency surgery for diverticular disease complicated by generalized and faecal peritonitis: a review. *Br J Surg* 1984; **71**:921–27.
18. Carr ND, Pullen BR, Hasleton PS, Schofield PF. Microvascular studies in human radiation bowel disease. *Gut* 1984; **25**:448–54.
19. Hatcher PA, Thomson HJ, Ludgate SN, Small WP, Smith AN. Surgical aspects of intestinal injury due to pelvic radiotherapy. *Ann Surg* 1985; **201**:470–75.

23

Infections of the uterus, vagina and tubes

Introduction

Community-acquired infections of the female genital tract are common but usually do not require the expertise of surgeons or gynaecologists for their diagnosis and treatment. Given adequate access to a good microbiological laboratory, there are few community-acquired infections which are not efficiently managed by general practitioners. There are, however, exceptions: biopsy may be required for the histological diagnosis of rare causes of vulvovaginitis; endomyometritis, salpingitis and pelvic peritonitis (often classed together as 'pelvic inflammatory disease') can cause severe illness, often mimicking other surgical conditions, and require a patient's admission to hospital.

Vulvovaginitis

One third of all women of child-bearing age suffer at some time in their lives from some form of vulvovaginitis. These infections cause much misery and occasionally serious septic complications. The vulva and vagina are lined by squamous epithelium which atrophies after the menopause and is then more vulnerable to infection. The internal milieu of the vagina is unique in harbouring, among numerous other organisms, a large number of lactobacilli which result in a pH of 3.8–4.2.

There are three common infections and several which are uncommon but potentially more dangerous. The common infections are Gardnerella, Trichomonas and Candida.

Gardnerella vaginitis

This acute infection encompasses most cases of 'non-specific vaginitis'. It is caused by the growth and invasion of a Gram-negative facultative anaerobic rod, formerly known as *Haemophilus vaginalis* but recognized in 1980 to belong to a new genus and renamed *Gardnerella vaginalis* to mark the valuable contributions to microbiology of Herman L. Gardner of Houston, Texas. The symptoms are of a malodorous vaginal discharge, and the diagnosis can be made with some confidence if the pH of the discharge is above 5 and no trichomonads are seen in an unstained slide of the fluid.

The culturing of *G. vaginalis* necessitates transporting the specimen in broth (such as Casman's broth with 5 per cent rabbit serum); optimal growth is on blood agar under an atmosphere of reduced oxygen and increased carbon dioxide. Gardner himself is doubtful of the contribution of *Bacteroides fragilis* acting synergistically with Gardnerella, but two facts suggest that *B. fragilis* may be involved – first the odour of the discharge, and secondly the response to metronidazole, which, in a dose of 500 mg twice daily orally or intravaginally for 7 days, is more effective than any antibiotic.[1] Intravaginal sulphonamides, povidone-iodine or chlorhexidine are sometimes used as adjuncts to metronidazole.

Trichomonas vaginitis

This protozoal infection is successfully treated by metronidazole. The organism is easily recognized on unstained wet films and, like *G. vaginalis*, is associated with a vaginal pH of more than 5. Metronidazole has rendered obsolete local treatment by aminacrine-sulphanilamide-allantoin (AVC) cream or pessaries;[2] topical antiseptics such as povidone-iodine and chlorhexidine may be useful adjuncts.

Candida vaginitis

In contrast to the other causes of vulvovaginitis, the incidence of vaginal thrush is increasing; this is associated with the increased use of broad-spectrum antibiotics and the widespread use of oral contraceptives. Diabetics and pregnant women are more susceptible to the disease.

Typical thrush patches on the vaginal wall are not often seen, but the characteristic branching fungus is easily distinguished microscopically in a wet film. In treatment oral or intravaginal nystatin is usually successful, but amphotericin or the newer imidazoles such as miconazole nitrate, clotrimazole, ketokonazole or econazole may be needed. Miconazole pessaries, tampons or cream or clotrimazole tablets or cream should be applied high in the vagina nightly for 6 days; in patients with recurrent candidiasis, twice-weekly application for several months is necessary.

Other causes of vulvovaginitis

Syphilis

It is easy to forget that a vulvo-vaginal ulcer can be a primary chancre. Dark-ground microscopy or later serology will establish the diagnosis, and treatment of the patient and her sexual partners by penicillin is essential. A single intramuscular injection of 2.4 million units (900 mg) of benzathene penicillin G, or eight daily injections of 0.6 million units (230 mg) of procaine penicillin G, appear to be equally effective.

Gonorrhoea

Primarily an endocervical infection, this usually presents with a vaginal discharge in the Gram-stained slide of which intracellular Gram-negative diplococci are seen. Treatment by a single dose of penicillin G is recommended; larger and larger doses have been needed as the years have passed, and there are now examples of plasmid-induced penicillin-resistant organisms which require a third generation cephalosporin to kill them.

Viral infections

Three distressing conditions are caused by viruses. Herpesvirus causes genital herpes, a recurrent painful eruption the attacks of which can sometimes be aborted by acyclovir cream. The infection can be transmitted to the newborn infant. Condyloma acuminatum is caused by the papillomavirus, and it may be associated with cervical dysplasia or even carcinoma. It sometimes responds to local application of 20 per cent podophyllin in tinct. benz. co. or 25 per cent ointment, but the lesions often require surgical destruction by cautery or cryocautery. Cryocautery is the preferred treatment for the third virus infection, molluscum contagiosum, which is caused by a poxvirus.

Secondary infections by mixed aerobic and anaerobic bacteria

A malodorous vaginal discharge may complicate carcinomas of the cervix or vagina, retained foreign bodies or senile atrophic vaginitis. In each case therapy is indicated for the underlying cause, but topical intravaginal application of metronidazole tablets and povidone-iodine gel will mitigate the symptoms.

Rare, mainly tropical, vulvovaginal infections

Granuloma inguinale, a chronic ulcerative condition associated with the presence of Donovan bodies in macrophages on microscopy, is caused by *Calymmatobacterium granulomatis*; this can be destroyed by many antibiotics, the preferred agent being doxycycline.

Chancroid is caused by *Haemophilus ducreyi*. The soft-based ulcer is often surrounded by satellite ulcers. It usually responds to sulphonamides with or without trimethoprim (sulphamethoxazole or co-trimoxazole); tetracycline is indicated if the sulphonamides fail to effect a cure. Lymphogranuloma inguinale, characterized by breaking down inguinal buboes, is caused by serotypes of *Chlamydia trachomatis*; it is diagnosed serologically, and treated by tetracycline.

Cutaneous amoebiasis, caused by *Entamoeba histolytica*, is recognized by microscopy and treated by metronidazole.

Staphylococcal toxic shock syndrome

This rare disease follows colonization of the vagina by a strain of *Staphylococcus aureus* which produces exotoxin C. It is usually associated with the use of 'superabsorbent' tampons. Admission to hospital for resuscitation is essential, and the preferred antimicrobial for first-line treatment is flucloxacillin given parenterally.

Pelvic inflammatory disease

This 'Pretty Inadequate Diagnosis' covers a large number of acute and chronic inflammatory conditions of the endometrium, salpinx and pelvic peritoneum. It is customary to separate these diseases into gonococcal and non-gonococcal, and in both there is a considerably higher incidence in patients who have had an intra-uterine contraceptive device inserted.[3] The aetiology is seldom monomicrobial, and anaerobic organisms (*Bacteroides* and *Peptococcus*) are often found in association with mixed aerobes. The conditions may be asymptomatic for long periods and then flare up into acute episodes of pain and fever.

Diagnosis

In young women the differentiation of salpingitis from appendicitis is difficult, and in doubtful cases it is better to remove a normal appendix than to allow a gangrenous appendix to perforate. There are no absolute guides to the differential diagnosis, but lower abdominal pain, vaginal discharge and fever should alert the surgeon, and the diagnosis is strengthened by the finding of greater tenderness on vaginal than on abdominal or rectal examination. Twenty minutes after a vaginal examination the patient's temperature will often be found to have risen considerably, presumably due to transient bacteraemia. Aerobic and anaerobic culture of the vaginal discharge or, (of greater value) of fluid aspirated by culdocentesis from the pouch of Douglas, allows an accurate aetiological diagnosis to be made and indicates the appropriate antibiotics. Grey scale ultrasound examination is non-invasive and, in the hands of a skilled technician, yields valuable information. Finally, examination under anaesthesia and laparoscopy should allow direct visualization of the tubes and should enable material to be taken for microbiological study.

Treatment

Systemic antibiotics are indicated. Until the microbiologist sends a report, the 'best buy' is metronidazole with a penicillin. If Gram-negative aerobes are cultured, it is likely that they will produce a beta-lactamase, and the penicillin should be changed to a more resistant antibiotic, for example amoxycillin-clavulanate or one of the cephalosporins. The antibiotics should be given parenterally during the acute phase of the illness; metronidazole may be given intravenously or in suppositories.

Operation is indicated in two circumstances – if the differential diagnosis from other causes of lower abdominal peritonitis cannot be made with confidence and, secondly, if a tubovarian abscess has ruptured and caused general peritonitis. The principles of pre- and postoperative management are no different from those of any laparotomy for peritonitis, which are considered in chapter 16. Postoperative complications are rare, and are also not specific to patients with pelvic inflammatory disease.

Septic abortion

One beneficial effect of the liberalization of abortion laws has been the steep decline in the number of admissions to hospital of young women with endomyometritis after 'back-street' abortions. Endomyometritis is a dangerous condition, frequently polymicrobial and accompanied by bacteraemia and septic shock. These patients require admission to hospital, resuscitation with oxygen inhalation and intravenous fluids, and combination antibiotic therapy with metronidazole (against anaerobes), ampicillin (against Gram-positive cocci) and a third generation cephalosporin (against beta-lactamase-producing Gram-negative enterobacteria). The occasional failure to respond rapidly to this regimen indicates the need for emergency hysterectomy.

Conclusions

Community-acquired infections of the female genital tract are commonly associated with sexual activity. They are caused by a large number of micro-organisms, prominent among which are those which are killed by metronidazole. This is probably the single most valuable antimicrobial in the gynaecological surgeon's armamentarium. Other useful agents are the penicillins, the imidazoles, the sulphonamides and the topical antiseptics povidone iodine and chlorhexidine. Surgical intervention is required mainly for the complications of pelvic inflammatory disease.

Further reading

Monif, GRG (ed). *Infectious Diseases in Obstetrics and Gynecology*. Second edition. Philadelphia, Harper and Row, 1982.

References

1. Spiegel CA, Amsel R, Eschenbach D, Schoenknecht F, Lolms KK. Anaerobic bacteria in non-specific vaginitis. *New Eng J Med* 1980; **303**:601–603.
2. Fleury FJ, van Bergen WS, Prentice RL, Russell JG, Singleton JA, Standard JV. Single dose of two grams of metronidazole for *Trichomonas vaginalis* infection. *Am J Obstet Gynecol* 1977; **128**:320–22.
3. Eschenbach DA. Epidemiology and diagnosis of acute pelvic inflammatory disease. *Obstet Gynecol* 1980; **55**(s):142–46.

24

Infections of the genito-urinary tract

The male genito-urinary tract is separated from any integument except at the external urinary meatus, and infections can therefore arise only by organisms ascending from this meatus or by blood-borne organisms. There are two principal defences against infection in these tracts: the first is the irrigating effect of freely-flowing urine, and the second is the integrity of the epithelial linings and the surface mucopolysaccharide on the bladder wall.[1] Infections in normal organs are uncommon; they are much more likely to complicate obstruction to the flow of urine or ulceration of the epithelium by stones or by cancer. I will consider infections associated with catheterization in Chapter 31.

Although most genito-urinary infections are caused by faecal Gram-negative rods (most often *Escherichia coli*), there are some which are caused by venereal organisms. Infection by *Mycobacterium tuberculosis* must also be considered, particularly in developing countries.

Venereal infections

Skin and lymph node infections

Syphilis, chancroid, lymphogranuloma venereum, granuloma inguinale, condyloma acuminatum and herpes simplex can all affect the skin of the glans penis, and may be accompanied by groin lymph node enlargement. Their differential diagnosis is important but it is seldom a surgical matter. I consider venereal and non-venereal female genital infections in Chapter 23.

Urethral infections

There are two microbial species which can adhere to and invade the urethral epithelium, and both species may spread from this epithelium to affect other parts of the genital system or even distant organs. They are *Neisseria gonorrhoeae* and *Chlamydia trachomatis*, the causes of gonococcal and non-gonococcal urethritis. The urethral discharge is purulent in the first infection and usually clear in the latter. The differentiation is made on Gram-stained smears of the discharge. The presence of characteristic Gram-negative intracellular cocci signifies infection with *N. gonorrhoeae*, their absence indicates infection with *C. trachomatis*. Treatment by penicillin for gonorrhoea, or tetracycline or co-trimoxazole for chlamydial infection, is usually successful, and the complications of urethral abscess or stricture are rare after gonorrhoea, unknown after non-specific urethritis. Systemic complications of non-gonococcal urethritis comprise Reiter's syndrome of ocular, arthritic and dermal lesions.

Non-venereal infections

Community-acquired infections of the bladder are common, particularly in young women and, if bladder emptying is efficient and there is no breach in the mucosa, these infections are effectively treated by antibacterial drugs. It is preferable to use specific narrow-spectrum non-antibiotic drugs such as naladixic acid or trimethoprim; the use of potent antibiotics carries with it the risk of disturbance of faecal ecology, diarrhoea and overgrowth of resistant bacteria.

Acute cystitis

The symptoms are frequency, dysuria, strangury and sometimes a little blood at the end of micturition. A clean specimen of urine should be examined by culture and by microsocopy of the centrifuged deposit. A colony count of more than 10^5 per ml, together with a neutrophil count of more than 5 per high power field, is significant.

Cystitis in children, in males of any age, and in women who fail to respond to appropriate chemotherapy, requires investigation of the possibility of an underlying cause – either an inefficiently emptying bladder or a lesion which breaches the mucosa. Physical examination may reveal a full bladder, an enlarged prostate or a hydronephrotic kidney. Ultrasound examination is important in detecting urinary retention or stones in kidneys or bladder, and intravenous urography supplements this examination. Finally, cystoscopy is essential to detect the presence of cancer, stones, foreign bodies or vesico-colic fistulae which disrupt the bladder mucosa.

Chronic cystitis

There are three conditions which lead to gross diminution in the capacity of the bladder and distressing frequency and dysuria. They are carcinomatous invasion of the bladder wall, diffuse tuberculous cystitis and chronic interstitial cystitis. The aetiology of chronic interstitial cystitis is ill-understood, and conservative treatment is mostly ineffectual. These patients require relief by enterocystoplasty together, if the interstitial fibrosis has caused ureteric obstruction, with re-implantation of the ureters.

Prostatitis

Sexually active men may complain of perineal aching, a reduction in the force of the stream of urine and perhaps a little blood at the beginning or end of micturition. Systematic symptoms of fever and rigors may signal an acute attack. Rectal examination reveals a tender, somewhat enlarged prostate and microscopic examination of the urine after prostatic massage reveals an excess of neutrophils and (usually) Gram-negative rods. Treatment of acute prostatitis by trimethoprim with or without sulphamethoxazole is usually effective, whereas the treatment of recurrent or chronic prostatitis is less effective and transurethral resection is disappointing, although Barnes and his colleagues reported better results by removing all prostatic tissue down to the capsule (radical transurethral resection of the prostate).[2]

Epididymo-orchitis

Most cases of epididymo-orchitis occur as complications of acute prostatitis, the organisms passing along the vasa or in the perivasal lymphatics to the epididymis. It used to be customary to divide and ligate both vasa during prostatectomy, but even this did not confer certain prophylaxis against the development of epididymitis, when prolonged urethral catheterization allowed infection of the lower urinary tract. Primary acute epididymitis is common in young men, and it may be mistaken for testicular torsion. It usually responds to antibiotic treatment but, particularly in old men, may go on to form an abscess which discharges through the scrotal skin.

Pyelonephritis

As in the bladder, so in the kidneys bacteria can only multiply and invade in the presence of urinary stasis and a breach in the transitional cell lining of the renal pelvis and calyces. Pyelonephritis is usually caused by the same Gram-negative rods which infect the bladder, but metastatic renal abscesses may result from bacteraemia and be caused by Gram-positive cocci or other organisms. Recurrent attacks of pyelonephritis may ultimately destroy the kidney and, if the condition is bilateral, are a potent cause of renal failure in young people.

Stasis of urine in the renal pelvis may be the result of congenital abnormalities in the bladder and urethra which interfere with efficient emptying of the bladder and allow reflux of infected urine up dilated ureters to the renal pelves. Acute pyelonephritis of pregnancy is more common on the right side, and it is associated with reversible hydronephrosis – more likely caused by hormones than by direct pressure of the pregnant uterus on the ureter.

Infections associated with renal calculi

Metabolic renal stones form in calyces, usually the lowermost, and often cause no complications or symptoms for years. If such a stone is discharged from the calyx, it may impact in the pelvi-ureteric junction or in the ureter, causing severe pain and obstruction which predisposes to infection. Intravenous urography will show delayed function of the affected kidney and dilatation above the stone. The attack usually settles with conservative treatment, including an appropriate antibacterial drug if there is evidence of infection. If the stone is not passed spontaneously, or if it is obviously too big to pass, it must be removed. A small stone in the lower ureter can often be extracted by a Dormia basket passed through an operating cystoscope, but bigger stones lying higher up require either open operation, percutaneous nephro-ureterolithotomy[3,4] or extracorporeal shockwave lithotripsy. The last technique is based on the Dornier lithotripter with the patient under general anaesthesia. Stones are fragmented into particles no larger than 2 mm in diameter which can be passed spontaneously. Early experience is favourable. Recurrent stone formation in the same calyx may be an indication for partial nephrectomy.

Perinephric abscess

Extension of infection from the renal pelvis into the perinephric fat is common, but rarely results in pus formation. If the infection is virulent enough, or the host defences sufficiently depressed, a perinephric abscess may form. Such a patient is ill, pyrexial and sometimes septicaemic. Tenderness and muscle rigidity usually prevent palpation of a mass, but ultrasound examination will reveal perinephric pus which must be drained. The kidney will usually have been damaged beyond repair and requires removal, either at the operation for drainage of the pus or later.

Tuberculous infections of the urinary tract

Mycobacterial bacteraemia may lead to the settling and proliferation of the organisms in a kidney, where they set up a typical abscess which ruptures into the pelvis and allows the spread of the disease down the ureter to the bladder and prostate, whence it may spread to the epididymis. The disease is recognized by the characteristic appearances in high-dose intravenous urograms in patients with 'sterile' pyuria. Cystoscopy may show a nonspecific inflammatory reaction surrounding a ureteric orifice, and prolonged culture of a fresh specimen of urine in a medium such as Lowenstein-Jensen's usually allows a definitive diagnosis.

Tuberculous pyelonephritis, cysto-prostatitis and epididymitis should be treated initially by a prolonged course of rifampicin 600 mg daily, together with isoniazid 300 mg daily and pyrazinamide 1 g daily. The urine should be kept acid by a daily dose of ascorbic acid 1 g. Surgical intervention is seldom required, the exceptions being nephrectomy for a totally destroyed kidney, caecocystoplasty for a contracted bladder, and epididymectomy for secondary infection of a discharging epididymitis.

References

1. Parsons CL, Shrom SH, Hanno PM, Mulholland SG. Bladder surface mucin. Examination of possible mechanisms for its antibacterial effect. *Invest Urol* 1978; **16**:196–99.
2. Barnes RW, Hadley HL, O'Donoghue EPN. Transurethral resection of the prostate for chronic bacterial prostatitis. *Prostate* 1982; **3**:215–19.
3. Wickham JEA. Percutaneous nephrolithotomy and lithotresis. Wickham JEA, Miller RA. (eds) *Percutaneous Renal Surgery*. Edinburgh, Churchill Livingstone, 1983, pp. 108–47.
4. Charig CR, Webb DR, Payne SR, Wickham JEA. Comparison of treatment of renal calculi by open surgery, percutaneous nephrolithotomy and extracorporeal shockwave lithotripsy. *Brit Med J* 1986; **292**:879–82.

25

Primary infections of bones and joints

Muscles, bones and joints are well away from any integument, and infections of these tissues arise in only three ways – through the blood stream as a complication of bacteraemia, by spread from infections in contiguous structures, or by direct breach of the overlying skin.

Myositis

Pyogenic myositis is rare except in some tropical countries, but secondary myositis may result from infections in adjacent structures, sometimes complicating osteomyelitis and (in the form of a psoas abscess) perforation of the appendix or colon. Treatment is required for the primary cause, together with drainage of abscesses.

Osteomyelitis

Pyogenic osteomyelitis differs from pyogenic infections elsewhere in the body in several ways. First, the inflammatory reaction confined by rigid bone can easily result in infarction of parts of the bone, and the formation of unabsorbable sequestra. Secondly, even apparent cure of the infection by a prolonged course of an appropriate antibiotic is no guarantee of lifelong immunity to recrudescences of infection. Finally, if the infection involves the epiphyseal plate of a growing long bone, either directly or by interference with its blood supply, serious deformity can result.

Acute haematogenous osteomyelitis

Although this is classically an infection with *Staphylococcus aureus* in the metaphyses of long bones in children, there are exceptions, and Gram-negative osteomyelitis and involvement of vertebral bodies can occur, particularly in adults and in any individual whose immune competence is depressed.

In children the diagnosis is made by the history of rapid onset of severe pain, usually around the knee or hip, with pyrexia, local swelling and tenderness. No radiographic abnormalities are seen in the early stages, but blood culture may reveal an organism. The child should be taken to the operating theatre as an emergency, and the suspected metaphysis drilled under general anaesthesia, both to provide material for microbiological examination and to relieve tension in the bone. Immediately after surgery the child should receive a methicillin such as flucloxacillin with a second antibiotic, fusidic acid being a common choice. If, as is usual, the organism is a penicillin-resistant but methicillin-sensitive *Staph aureus*, this regimen should be continued for at least 3 weeks. If a different bacterial species is isolated, the antibiotics should be changed to more appropriate ones. Properly treated it is unusual for acute haematogenous osteomyelitis to proceed to chronic osteomyelitis.

Acute haematogenous vertebral osteomyelitis

These infections are rare. They occur in adults, and the patient presents with backache and general illness. About half the cases are caused by *Staph aureus*, the rest are caused by Gram-negative organisms of which the commonest are *Escherichia coli* and *Proteus* species.[1] The diagnosis may easily be overlooked unless a technetium bone scan is done. Needle aspiration of the affected vertebral body should be performed to obtain samples for microbiological examination, and appropriate antibiotics should be given for at least 1 month.

Osteitis pubis

This is an uncommon complication of operations on the bladder and is usually caused by infection in the retropubic space by Gram-negative aerobic organisms, of which perhaps the most difficult to eradicate is *Pseudomonas aeruginosa*. The patient presents with pain, radiographic signs in the anterior pubic rami are seen, and the treatment is by a course of an appropriate antibiotic which should be continued for several weeks.

Other examples of osteomyelitis from contiguous infections

Osteomyelitis of phalanges or metacarpals is an occasional complication of neglected pulp space infections, infected puncture wounds on the sole of the foot, or infective – often diabetic – gangrene. Both antibiotics and operation are indicated. Postoperative wound infection after lower limb amputations for gangrene may spread to the divided bone, resulting in a sequestrum and a discharging sinus until the sequestrum is removed.

Acute osteomyelitis following compound fractures

It is rare for infection to follow timely treatment of a compound fracture by parenteral antibiotics, debridement and skin closure. Nevertheless, of all causes of acute osteomyelitis, compound fractures and open plating, and pinning or screwing of simple fractures are probably the most common. Treatment demands antibiotics, removal of the hardware from the bones, debridement of dead bone and external fixation in a Denham frame, or equivalent apparatus, often for several months.

Chronic osteomyelitis

Any variety of acute osteomyelitis can become chronic, and the lesion is unique in that the clinical symptoms and signs may be delayed for years after apparent cure of the acute condition. Occasionally, a chronic abscess cavity referred to as a Brodie's abscess can be the presenting feature. Pain, swelling and sinuses, as well as pyrexia and general ill health, are features of chronic osteomyelitis, and radiography always shows some abnormality, ranging from areas of translucency with periosteal new bone formation to sequestra.

Antibiotics alone, even if they are specific for the usually mixed bacterial flora involved, are not enough for cure which demands in addition operation with debridement of dead tissue, saucerization of bone and primary skin cover. There is a place for postoperative antibiotic irrigation–suction through one or more fine-bore polyethylene catheters, and excellent results have attended the use of strings of polymethylmethacrylate beads incorporating gentamicin.[2] These beads are left in contact with the infected bone after debridement and are removed at a second operation after several weeks, during which time gentamicin has gradually leached out of the beads.

When chronic osteomyelitis follows either a compound fracture or an open operation for a simple fracture of a long bone, it is usually accompanied by non-union of the fracture, and the treatment involves not only the control of the infection but also, subsequently, the insertion of cancellous bone grafts coupled with rigid external fixation.[3]

Osteomyelitis caused by specific microorganisms

Osseous gummas of tertiary syphilis are so rare that surgeons tend to forget their possibility. They present with swelling surrounding a cavity in a long bone and frequently break through the skin, establishing a typical 'punched out' ulcer. The disease is amenable to penicillin treatment.

Actinomycosis of the jaw ('lumpy jaw') is less likely to be overlooked when it presents with multiple sinuses discharging 'sulphur granules'. It is usually cured by 3 months of penicillin.

Tuberculous osteomyelitis is almost exclusively a disease of vertebral bodies, causing collapse of these bones, kyphosis and sometimes paraplegia from pressure on the spinal cord. Most patients without neurological signs do well with bed-rest on a hard (sometimes a plaster of Paris) bed and 2 years of combination antituberculous chemotherapy. The presence of neurological signs which do not clear up after a week or two of this regimen is an indication for spinal cord decompression by debridement of cold abscesses and granulation tissue, followed by spinal fusion.

Septic arthritis

Acute haematogenous arthritis is rare. Any joint may be affected, but the disease attacks most often the knee, hip or shoulder. *Staph aureus* is by far the most frequently isolated pathogen but, particularly in sick people whose immune competence is subnormal, other bacteria including aerobic and anaerobic Gram-negative rods may be involved. *Neisseria gonorrhoeae* is a rare cause.

The disease presents with a painful, swollen joint, usually with systemic illness. Aspiration of joint fluid or open or arthroscopic biopsy of synovial membrane is essential for identification of the causative organism, and an appropriate antibiotic regimen should be instituted for at least 4 weeks. If the diagnosis has been delayed sufficiently to allow destruction of joint surfaces, operation should be undertaken to remove dead tissue. The results of early antibiotic treatment are good, but destruction of articular cartilage leaves a joint which is painful and with limited movement. Late arthrodesis or joint replacement may be required.

Other causes of joint infections

Penetrating trauma, particularly if a foreign body is implanted in the joint, may be followed by joint sepsis if early debridement is not carried out. Tuberculous arthritis, usually of the hip, is rare in Western countries but an important cause of disablement in the Third World. Early destruction of the articular surfaces is usual, and complete functional recovery with antituberculous chemotherapy is exceptional.

Finally, probably the most important cause of septic arthritis in developed countries is deep infection of total joint arthroplasties. Although in the best centres this involves less than 1 per cent of all replacement arthroplasties, it is nevertheless a common condition, and the average surgeon is more likely to encounter iatrogenic than community-acquired joint sepsis.

References

1. Anonymous. Pyogenic infections of the spine. *Lancet* 1985; i:619–20.
2. Grieben A. Results of Septopal in more than 1500 cases of bone and soft tissue infections: a review of clinical trials. *J Bone Joint Surg* 1980; 62B:275–76.
3. Fitzgerald RH Jr, Kelly PJ. Infections of the skeletal system. In: Simmons RL, Howard RJ (eds). *Surgical Infectious Diseases*. New York, Appleton-Century-Crofts, 1982, pp. 1005–1028.

Part V

Hospital-acquired Surgical Infections

26

Exogenous operating-theatre-acquired infections

Infections in lungs, bladder and blood-stream may be caused by the invasive techniques which are required during major surgical operations. It is, however, almost impossible to determine their precise pathogenesis and to place responsibility firmly on operating theatre processes as opposed to those processes involved in postoperative ward care. I propose considering these nosocomial infections in the section on ward-acquired infections.

Surgical wound infections are, however, amenable to classification into operating-theatre-acquired and ward-acquired. In both cases the role of host defences against contaminating bacteria is important. I have called operating-theatre-acquired wound infection 'primary' and ward-acquired infection 'secondary'.[1] Their end results are identical, and the distinction cannot usually be made on microbiological grounds. Clinically, however, the distinction is easy. I will define these two entities but postpone further discussion on secondary wound infection.

Definition of wound infection

Most workers adopt Ljungqvist's simple definition 'a clear collection of pus, which empties itself spontaneously or after incision'.[2] It is not always quite as clear-cut. I regard any wound which discharges fluid containing bacteria, other than the patient's own normal skin flora, as infected. I classify wound infections as either major, which cause constitutional disturbances (notably pyrexia) and delay patients' release from hospital, or minor, which do neither.

Wilson and his colleagues devised a more complicated scoring system for cardio-thoracic operations to which they gave the name ASEPSIS.[3] A is for additional treatment and they score 5 for drainage under local anaesthetic, 10 for debridement under general anaesthetic and 10 for antibiotic prescription. For the following four (SEPS) they estimate the length of wound affected during the first 5 days after operation and score accordingly; Serous discharge and Erythema score 1 for 20 per cent affected, up to 5 for 100 per cent, whereas Purulent exudate and Separation of deep tissues score 2 for 20 per cent affected up to 10 for 100 per cent. Finally, Isolation of bacteria scores 10 and Stay as an in-patient prolonged over 14 days scores 5. They regard a score of 0–10 as satisfactory healing, 11–20 as disturbed healing and over 20 as wound infection, 21–30 being minor, 31–40 moderate, and over 40 as severe.

Secondary wound infection

A dry closed wound is immune to bacterial invasion within a few hours and, if such a wound discharges pus, the contamination has nearly always occurred in the operating theatre.[4] If, however, the wound discharges blood, serum or lymph, if an open drain is led through the wound, if the skin edges of the wound die because of a poor blood supply, or if a fistula discharges through the wound, then exogenous or endogenous bacteria may colonize and invade. The contaminating organisms are commonly *Staphylococcus aureus*, but contamination of weeping groin wounds is often by the patient's own Gram-negative bacteria.

Primary wound infection after clean operations

Unless the operation involves an incision into tissues containing bacteria, any organisms landing on the wound where they can multiply and invade arise from exogenous sources. These include surgical instruments and swabs, the hands of the operating team, the skin of the patient and the air of the operating theatre.

Sterilization of instruments and swabs

The application of steam under pressure is the best method of sterilizing instruments and dressings. It is customary nowadays for sets of instruments and dressings to be placed on stainless steel trays which are then double-wrapped in cotton cloth or paper and sterilized in autoclaves. There are, however, some materials which are destroyed by high temperature steam sterilization, and for these the choice is between gamma irradiation and the use of antiseptic chemicals. Disposable polyethylene syringes and needles which have plastic hubs are sterilized by gamma rays, as are vascular prostheses (although these can be autoclaved). Ethylene oxide gas is an efficient chemical method of sterilization but combines with rubber and, unless the instrument is allowed to breathe off the gas, it can be toxic to human tissues. Activated glutaraldehyde is a reasonable alternative for instruments such as flexible endoscopes, but the instrument must first be thoroughly cleaned of organic matter and then the channels irrigated with glutaraldehyde before being rinsed with sterile water and dried.[5]

Sterilization of the hands of the operating team

The demonstration that exogenous infections of wounds (including the uterus during childbirth) can be reduced by chemically disinfecting the operator's hands predates the recognition of the role of bacteria. Both Semmelweis and Oliver Wendell Holmes showed that the hands of accoucheurs were the principal carriers of puerperal sepsis, and Semmelweis reduced the death rate at the Allgemeines Krankenhaus in Vienna from 11.4 per cent in 1846 to 1.3 per cent in 1848 by insisting that accoucheurs' hands should be washed in chloride of lime before examining women in labour.

The universal adoption of sterile surgical gloves by the operating team is a relatively modern development and resulted from Halsted's concern for the hands of his operating theatre nurse.[6,7] She could not use the corrosive sublimate, which customarily followed soap and water cleansing, without developing severe dermatitis. Halsted wrote to the Goodyear Rubber Company and asked them to make rubber gloves for the nurse's protection. These were successful and were soon used by all surgeons, although there is no evidence that they reduce the risks of wound infection, the incidence of which is no higher in clean operations when the gloves have been punctured during the operation.[8]

The ritual of the 'surgical scrub' is still observed in some parts of the world – the hands and forearms are scrubbed with a nailbrush with soap and running water for 10 minutes before each operation. This ritual ignores the fact, known for 50 years, that the microflora of the skin of the hands comprises not only transient pathogens which have been acquired by contact with contaminated substances and which are easily removed by a 30-second wash with a chlorhexidine or povidone iodine detergent and water, but also the resident microflora, mainly coagulase-negative staphylococci and coryne-bacteria, which are easily removed from the surface of the skin but which reside also in the depths of the skin glands and rise from there to the surface.

Lowbury and his colleagues wrote extensively on the subject of suitable hand disinfectants.[9] They concluded that a 2-minute wash (after brush-cleaning of the nails) with 4 per cent chlorhexidine detergent followed by drying on a sterile towel and then the application of 10 ml of 70 per cent alcoholic chlorhexidine, which is allowed to dry on the skin, not only achieves 99 per cent sterility but also has a residual antibacterial action lasting several hours. This is my practice before the first operation in a session. I do not remove gloves and gown at the end of an operation, but aseptically before the next case. I then apply alcoholic chlorhexidine to my hands and forearms before donning fresh sterile gown and gloves.

Sterilization of the skin of the patient

The same considerations apply to the skin of the patient at the site of incision. My own preference in abdominal and groin operations is alcoholic iodine, for other operations I prefer alcoholic chlorhexidine. Four other aspects must also be considered – pre-operative shaving, length of stay in hospital before operation, pre-operative whole-body disinfection, and adhesive incise drapes.

Pre-operative shaving

In his extensive audit of the incidence of wound infection, Cruse found that patients whose abdomens were shaved the day before abdominal operations were more likely to suffer a wound infection than those who were either not shaved, shaved immediately before operation, or had hairs removed by a depilatory cream.[10]

Prolonged pre-operative hospital stay

Patients exposed to hospital pathogens for more than 24 hours are at greater risk of developing wound infections.[11] So many factors concerning host defences are involved that it is difficult to isolate prolongation of hospital stay *per se* as the cause of the increased incidence of wound infection. My preference on both economic and scientific grounds is to complete pre-operative investigations and treatments before admitting patients to hospital for elective operations, and then to operate within 24 hours.

Pre-operative whole-body patient disinfection

Brandberg and his colleagues showed in a non-randomized trial that pre-operative showering with a chlorhexidine detergent reduced the surface counts of skin bacteria and the incidence of groin wound infections to 8.0 per cent from 17.5 per cent in controls.[12] These results were not substantiated by Ayliffe and his colleagues who found no significant improvement in the rate of wound infection from pre-operative chlorhexidine-detergent bathing in 5536 patients undergoing clean or clean-contaminated operations.[13]

Adhesive incise drapes

Theoretically, isolation of the skin in the vicinity of an incision should reduce the risks of wound contamination by skin bacteria. Lilly and his colleagues, however concluded that 'Adhesive drapes probably give no protection against bacterial contamination of operation wounds'.[14] Controlled clinical trials both in my unit[15] and elsewhere have failed to show any benefit in terms of wound infection rates from the use of these drapes. A medicated incise drape (Ioban) has been introduced but has not yet been sufficiently evaluated.

The special case of operations involving prosthetic implants

In general surgery the resident skin flora is of such low pathogenicity that its importance is overwhelmed by that of endogenous pathogens. When, however, prostheses are inserted into the heart, arteries, brain or joints, even minor contamination with *Staph. epidermidis* can result in disastrous infection, and it is in these operations that two extra preventive measures have been suggested – sterilization of the air of the operating theatre, and pre- or peroperative administration of an effective antibiotic.[16]

Many strains of coagulase-negative staphylococci are resistant to methicillin and to third-generation cephalosporins, and cardiac surgeons often prescribe gentamicin in addition to flucloxacillin for prophylaxis in prosthetic valve operations. If resistant staphylcocci are a problem vancomycin or rifampicin should be used instead.[17]

In coronary bypass operations the main infective complication at a London hospital was found to be sternal wound infection, which occurred in 8.7 per cent of 309 operations.[18] This was almost certainly the result of the harvesting of the saphenous vein, half the species recovered being of skin origin and half of intestinal origin.

An important variant on antibiotics in prosthetic surgery has been the use of bone cement (polymethylmethacrylate) incorporating gentamicin in joint replacement operations[19,20] and the bonding of oxacillin to vascular prostheses. Oxacillin bonding has not yet been evaluated clinically.

Sterilization of the air in the operating theatre

The air is sterile in an unoccupied operating theatre ventilated at positive pressure with filtered air. It is when people come in and move about that bacterial contamination by coagulase-negative staphylococci and diphtheroids occurs. The bacteria are attached to skin squames with a diameter of approximately 25 mm and a thickness of 3–5 mm. The role of droplet or nasal contamination of the air has not been established, and the traditional surgical mask is probably quite unnecessary. There are two rules which should always be applied, and four other techniques which may have a role in the prevention of deep wound infection in patients having prosthetic implants. The two simple rules are as follows:

- Exclude from the operating theatre any person who has an active skin infection.
- Make sure that as few people as possible come into the operating theatre.

It is customary for people going into an operating theatre to discard their street clothes and don clean cotton shirt, trousers and shoes. This probably serves no purpose other than ensuring that the operating theatre does not become a committee room.

The four techniques which have sound theoretical bases but whose cost-benefit is more equivocal are the wearing of non-woven or close-woven impermeable clothing, laminar flow ventilation, the total isolation of the patient in a ventilated plastic tent and ultraviolet irradiation of the theatre.

Normal cotton shirts, trousers and surgical gowns can breathe, which makes them comfortable but also allows egress of infected skin squames, particularly when the clothes are moist. It is perfectly easy to make clothing of material which is impermeable to bacteria, but the wearer soon becomes uncomfortably hot unless the suit is exhaust-ventilated.

As for laminar flow as opposed to plenum ventilation, vertically-directed flow has been shown to be more efficient than horizontally-directed flow in keeping the site of the wound free from aerial contamination.[21,22] The Medical Research Council set up a controlled clinical trial in 8055 joint replacement operations, randomizing them to be performed in theatres which were either plenum or laminar flow ventilated. The trial demonstrated that the air in laminar flow ventilated theatres yielded 6.5 colony-forming units/m^3, compared with 161 cfu/m^3 in plenum-ventilated theatres,[23] and subsequently revealed that the rate of deep infection was 3.4 per cent in patients who were not given prophylactic antibiotics and were operated on in plenum ventilated theatres, compared with 1.2 per cent in patients not given antibiotics and operated on in laminar flow ventilated theatres.[24] On the other hand, when patients were given prophylactic antibiotics the rates of deep infection between the two ventilation systems (0.8 per cent and 0.3 per cent respectively) did not differ significantly.

The use of a whole-body isolator in which the patient lies, the surgeon operating through sleeves, ensures the kind of absolute sterility which is necessary in some microbiological and pharmaceutical processes.[25] It is, however, cumbersome and has not attracted many adherents.

Finally, ultraviolet irradiation of the operating theatre has fallen into disfavour, and it was shown by a Committee of the National Research Council to produce only marginal benefit.[11]

References

1. Pollock AV. Surgical wound sepsis. *Lancet* 1979; ii:1283–86.
2. Ljungqvist U. Wound sepsis after clean operations. *Lancet* 1964; i:1095–97.
3. Wilson APR, Treasure T, Sturridge MF, Gruneberg RN. A scoring system (ASEPSIS) for postoperative wound infections for use in clinical trials of antibiotic prophylaxis. *Lancet* 1986; i:311–13.
4. Schauerhamer RA, Edlich RF, Panek P, Thul J, Prusak M, Wangensteen OH. Studies in the management of the contaminated wound. VII Susceptibility of surgical wounds to postoperative surface contamination. *Am J Surg* 1971; 122:74–7.
5. O'Connor HJO, Axon ATR. Gastrointestinal endoscopy: infection and disinfection. *Gut* 1983; 24:1067–77.
6. Wangensteen OH, Wangensteen SD, Klinger CF. Some pre-Listerian and post-Listerian antiseptic wound practices and the emergence of asepsis. *Surg Gynecol Obstet* 1973; 137:677–702.
7. Proskauer C. Development and use of the rubber glove in surgery and gynecology. *J Hist Med* 1958; 13:373–81.
8. Davidson AIG, Clark C, Smith G. Postoperative wound infection: a computer analysis. *Br J Surg* 1971; 58:333–37.
9. Lilly HA, Lowbury EJL, Wilkins MD. Limits to progressive reduction of resident skin bacteria by disinfection. *J Clin Path* 1979; 32:382–85.
10. Cruse PJE, Foord R. The epidemiology of wound infection. A 10-year prospective study of 62,939 wounds. *Surg Clin N Am* 1980; 60:27–40.
11. Report of an *ad hoc* Committee on Trauma, Division of Medical Sciences, National Academy of Sciences – National Research Council. Postoperative wound infections. The influence of ultraviolet irradiation of the operating room and of various other factors. *Ann Surg* 1964; 160 (Suppl):1–192.
12. Brandberg A, Andersson I. In: Maibach H, Aly R. (eds) *Skin Microbiology: Relevance to Clinical Infection*. New York, Springer Verlag, 1981, pp. 92–96 and 98–102.
13. Ayliffe GAJ, Noy MF, Babb JR, Davies JG, Jackson J. A comparison of preoperative bathing with chlorhexidine-detergent and non-medicated soap in the prevention of wound infection. *J Hosp Infect* 1983; 4:237–44.
14. Lilly HA, London PS, Lowbury EJL, Porter MF. Effects of adhesive drapes on contamination of operation wounds. *Lancet* 1970; ii:431–32.
15. Jackson DW, Pollock AV, Tindal DS. The use of a plastic adhesive drape in the prevention of wound infection. *Br J Surg* 1971; 58:340–42.
16. Anonymous. Coagulase-negative staphylococci. *Lancet* 1981; i:139–40.
17. Anonymous. Antibiotic cover for cardiac surgery. *Lancet* 1985; ii:701–702.
18. Farrington M, Webster M, Fenn A, Phillips I. Study of cardiothoracic wound infection at St. Thomas' Hospital. *Br J Surg* 1985; 72:759–62.
19. Elson RA, Jephcott AE, McGechie DB, Verettas D. Antibiotic-loaded acrylic cement. *J Bone Joint Surg* 1977; 59B:200–205.
20. Greco RS, Harvey RA. The role of antibiotic bonding in the prevention of

vascular prosthetic infections. *Ann Surg* 1982; **195**:168–71.
21. Howarth FH. Prevention of airborne infection during surgery. *Lancet* 1985; i:386–88.
22. Bechtol CO. Environmental bacteriology in the unidirectional (vertical) operating room. *Arch Surg* 1979; **114**:784–88.
23. Lowbury EJL, Lidwell OM. Multi-hospital trial on the use of ultraclean air systems in orthopaedic operating rooms to reduce infection: preliminary communication. *J Roy Soc Med* 1978; **71**:800–806.
24. Lidwell OM, Lowbury EJL, Whyte W, Blowers R, Stanley SJ, Lowe D. Effect of ultraclean air in operating rooms on deep sepsis in the joint after total hip or knee replacement: a randomized study. *Br Med J* 1982; **285**:10–14.
25. McLauchlan J, Pilcher MF, Trexler PC, Whalley RC. The surgical insulator. *Br Med J* 1974; i:322–24.

27

Endogenous operating-theatre-acquired infections

It is the surgical wound itself which is at greatest risk of infection from endogenous bacterial contamination during operations. Although the same bacteria may contaminate the peritoneum or pleura, these cavities are normally so well provided with defensive mechanisms that it takes a much larger inoculum of pathogenic organisms to cause peritonitis or empyema than it does to cause wound infection. The occurrence of peritonitis after a clean-contaminated or even a contaminated operation nearly always means the failure of an internal suture line, and I will consider this complication in Chapter 32.

Detection of visceral and parietal bacterial contamination

Major operations upset the host's defences. Not only can humoral and cellular mechanisms be depressed, but local defects arise including anoxia, ill-vascularized fatty tissue, dead tissue and foreign bodies such as sutures. In these circumstances it takes only a small inoculum of bacteria to cause infection in a surgical wound. The detection of this contamination during operation demands special microbiological techniques, particularly related to the taking and transporting of specimens. If a swab is applied to even a heavily contaminated viscus (e.g. the inside of the colon), placed in a sterile cardboard tube and sent at the end of the operating list to the Department of Microbiology, there is a strong chance that agar plate cultures will show no growth. Welbourn and his colleagues found that 21 out of 31 swabs of faeces in patients prepared for two days with neomycin, bacitracin and nystatin, yielded no growth.[1] We now know that colonic contents are never sterile, whatever the preparation.

In the Veterans Administration trial of neomycin/erythromycin base preparation for elective colorectal operations,[2] culture of the fluid obtained by wound irrigation with 10 ml of Ringer lactate gave disappointing results; only 25 out of 91 wound irrigation fluid samples yielded intestinal organisms, and there was no correlation between the detection of contamination and subsequent wound infection, which developed in 17 per cent of patients with positive cultures and 18 per cent of those with negative cultures.

Thioglycollate agar transport medium is widely used for the transport of swabs from the operating theatre or wards to the Department of Microbiology. It is adequate in allowing the detection of gross bacterial contamination, but is much less sensitive than immediate culture in an enrichment broth. Anyone who attempted to define bacteraemia by dipping a swab in blood and transporting it in thioglycollate medium would be derided; blood cultures only give acceptable information if the sample of blood is immediately placed in nutrient broth and incubated, species identification being made by subsequent subculture on agar plates. Stone and his colleagues placed visceral and parietal swabs in peptone broth during abdominal operations to define operative bacterial contamination.[3] They showed that wound cultures yielding two or more species of intestinal organisms predicted a significantly higher rate of wound infection than those yielding one species, which in turn predicted a higher rate than those which were sterile.

We have compared the sensitivity and predictive value of parietal swabs transported in thioglycollate medium with duplicate swabs immediately placed in cooked meat broth and incubated in the operating theatre suite before being sent to the Department of Microbiology for aerobic and anaerobic subculture.[4] The study involved 817 emergency and elective abdominal operations, and the results are summarized in Table 27.1. The cooked meat broth cultures were significantly more sensitive in detecting parietal contamination ($P < 0.001$), and the finding of a sterile wound culture was significantly more likely to predict healing without wound infection ($P = 0.007$). We confirmed Stone's finding that the identification of two or more species of intestinal organisms in the broth cultures of parietal swabs predicted a significantly higher rate of wound infection than the isolation of one species alone.

Bacterial burden of the abdominal hollow viscera

There is an enormous difference between the bacterial content of the biliary-pancreatic and urinary systems which are always sterile unless diseased, the stomach, duodenum and jejunum in which there are few potential pathogens, the ileum in which are small numbers of enterobacteriaceae, and the colon which is colonized by vast numbers of aerobic and anaerobic bacteria, the principal species being *Escherichia coli*, enterococci and *Bacteroides*. Staphylococci and yeasts also are often isolated.

Infections of the biliary-pancreatic and urinary systems are nearly always by aerobic enterobacteriaceae or enterococci, anaerobic infection being rare.

Prevention of endogenous bacterial contamination of surgical wounds

Evacuation of the infective contents of hollow viscera

Although this principle applies mainly to the colon, it is nevertheless sensible to ensure that any viscus which one incises or excises shall be as empty as possible. The stomach can be emptied by a nasogastric (or large-bore orogastric) tube, the bladder by a catheter, the small intestine by withholding solid food for 24 hours before elective operations, and the oesophagus by pre-operative oesophagoscopy and aspiration of the contents.

It is easy, by any one of a number of techniques, to empty an unobstructed colon. It is when there is partial or complete obstruction of the colon that difficulties arise.

Table 27.1 Wound infections in 817 abdominal operations – correlation with two methods of transporting swabs

	Thioglycollate medium			Cooked meat broth		
	Total	Total wound infection (%)	Major wound infection (%)	Total	Total wound infection (%)	Major wound infection (%)
Both visceral and parietal swab sterile*	380	13 (3.4)	0	369	14 (3.9)	0
Visceral swab contaminated, parietal swab sterile*	301	57 (18.9)	3 (1.0)	193	19 (9.8)	0
Single pathogenic species in parietal swab	105	48 (45.7)	11 (10.5)	146	48 (32.9)	7 (4.8)
Two or more pathogenic species in parietal swab	31	15 (48.4)	4 (12.9)	109	52 (47.7)	11 (10.1)
Total	817	133 (16.3)	18 (2.2)	817	133 (16.3)	18 (2.2)

* 'Sterile' includes skin flora

Evacuation of the unobstructed colon

Whatever method one selects it is sensible to restrict the patient's oral intake to clear fluids for 24 hours before operation. The options are to administer either aperients or enemas and colonic washouts (or both). The choice must be made not only on grounds of efficiency but also of acceptability to patients. Until 10 years ago my patients were prepared by repeated oral administration of 30 ml of 50 per cent magnesium sulphate solution on the 2 pre-operative days. This was effective but the taste was resented. I then adopted whole gut irrigation, which involved the introduction through a nasogastric tube of up to 10 litres of salt solution in 2 hours while the patient sat on a toilet seat. The results were satisfactory but the method was unacceptable to many patients. I tried Picolax (13 g magnesium citrate with 10 g sodium picosulphate), giving two sachets three times on the day before operation. This I found not quite as effective as the previous methods. I have now standardized on mannitol, giving 100 g in 1 litre of water by mouth on the day before operation followed by 2 litres of any clear fluid by mouth, or of Ringer lactate solution intravenously. I find this cleanses the unobstructed bowel and is tolerable to patients. It does, however, allow increased bacterial production of hydrogen and methane in the colon and should not be given if diathermy is to be used during the resection.

Evacuation of the obstructed colon

Even incomplete colonic obstruction will thwart attempts to empty the bowel by the oral administration of aperients, and may precipitate complete obstruction. In these cases it is better to avoid aperients altogether and to concentrate on evacuation of the distal colon by enemas and washouts. A technique which I find valuable in allowing primary anastomosis, after resection of obstructing left-sided colonic lesions, is peroperative orthograde lavage.[5] A Foley catheter is introduced into the caecum either through the stump of the appendix or through a stab in the terminal ileum. It is connected to a reservoir of tap water. Once the obstructing lesion has been resected the colon is intubated between clamps with a 1.5 metre length of 4 cm sterile corrugated polyvinyl tube (anaesthetic scavenger tubing serves well). This is led into a container on the floor and the colon washed out with tap water.The lavage may require as much as 10 litres of tap water and considerable massage of the colon by the surgeon. It is my practice to add 100 ml of aqueous povidine iodine to the last litre: work from Condon's unit showed that intralumenal povidone iodine is capable of substantially reducing the bacterial burden of the colon in dogs within 20 minutes.[6]

Reducing the concentration of bacteria in the contents of hollow viscera

For practical purposes this applies only to the colon although it is prudent, if time allows, to give pre-operative systemic antimicrobials in an attempt to sterilize other hollow viscera which are normally sterile but which are infected because of disease.

I must emphasize that the colon cannot be sterilized; its bacterial content can merely be reduced. The history of antimicrobial bowel preparation starts with the introduction of sulphanilamide. Garlock and Seley prepared 21 patients with oral sulphanilamide 1 g 4-hourly for 3 days.[7] They had previously found the predominant colonic organism to be a haemolytic streptococcus, but in the prepared patients they were not able to isolate this organism from the colon. Poth introduced two non-absorbable sulphonamides – succinylsulphathiazole and phthalylsulphathiazole;[8] the use of the latter became standard practice for 30 years. Phthalylsulphathiazole is probably more effective than neomycin: one of the first random control trials was in Goligher's unit.[9] He and his co-workers randomized 150 patients about to undergo elective colorectal operations to receive 5 days of mechanical bowel preparation only (group 1), or combined with 5 days of phthalylsulphathiazole (group 2) or with 2 days of phthalylsulphathiazole together with neomycin (group 3). They withdrew 22 patients and reported anastomotic leak rates of 52 per cent, 24 per cent and 22 per cent and abdominal wound infection rates of 40 per cent, 26 per cent and 20 per cent respectively. They concluded that the addition of neomycin to phthalylsulphathiazole did not improve the results of the sulphonamide alone.

Modern methods of antibacterial bowel cleansing stem from the acknowledgement of the pathogenic potential of intestinal anaerobes. A random control trial was published from the Mayo Clinic in 1974.[10] These workers randomized 196 patients about to undergo elective colorectal operations to receive, during the 48 hours before operation, oral neomycin alone, oral neomycin with tetracycline, or placebo. Neomycin alone resulted in a wound infection rate of 41 per cent, not significantly different from the placebo rate of 43 per cent. Combination antibiotic preparation reduced the wound infection rate to 5 per cent.

A publication which has had a great influence on current surgical practice in the USA is the Veterans Administration placebo-controlled trial of three pre-operative doses, starting 19 hours before operation, of oral neomycin with erythromycin base.[11] Of the 56 patients receiving the antibiotics, five suffered wound infections (8.9 per cent) compared with 21 of the 60 patients (35 per cent) in the placebo group. All other infective complications were reduced by the antimicrobial preparation.

The remarkable ability of metronidazole (and tinidazole) to kill anaerobic bacteria while having no effect on aerobic organisms was reported by Tally in 1972.[12] Its clinical application to colorectal surgery was, however, delayed until 1975 when Goldring and his colleagues reported a wound infection rate of 8 per cent in 25 patients given pre-operative oral kanamycin and metronidazole for 3 days compared with 44 per cent in 25 controls.[13] Since that time the standard antimicrobial bowel preparation in Britain has been by an oral aminoglycoside together with metronidazole, although most surgeons have reduced the duration of preparation to 24 hours. There have been few attempts to compare the neomycin/erythromycin base regimen with the aminoglycoside/metronidazole regimen. An exception is from my department.[14] We found a significantly greater proportion of infective events (abdominal and perineal wound infections, peritonitis and anastomotic dehiscences) in the erythromycin group than in the group given metronidazole.

Measures to prevent spill of the contents of hollow viscera

No surgeon will condone, if it can be avoided, overt spillage of the contents of a viscus which he is incising or excising. Such avoidance involves standard surgical techniques of clamps, suction and swabbing. A special variation on this theme is the use of the so-called closed intestinal anastomosis. This technique allows only brief access of the contents of the intestine to the wound, but the results appear to be no different from those achieved by the more usual open techniques.

Measures to prevent access to the wound by the contents of hollow viscera

Generations of abdominal surgeons have attempted to isolate the wound from potential endogenous bacterial contamination by inserting 'lap pads' tucked into the peritoneal cavity. The modern development of this idea has been the use of a plastic ring drape.[15] We have shown, however (unpublished observations), that it is impossible to remove the drape without contaminating the wound and controlled trials in my unit and elsewhere[16,17] failed to show a reduction in wound infection rates in patients in whom the drape was used. We attempted to improve the technique by constructing cloth ring drapes which were soaked in aqueous povidone iodine solution or, later, chlorhexidine solution. We showed, however, that, although these antiseptic wound guards reduced the incidence of parietal contamination, they had only a marginal influence on the rates of wound infection.[18, 19]

Prevention of infection if contamination is inevitable

Contamination of a surgical wound by pathogenic bacteria is one ingredient in the development of infection, the occurrence of which, however, is determined by the adequacy of the local and general host defence mechanisms. Burke referred to the work of Sir Ashley Miles, summing it up as 'If the host is not susceptible to bacterial invasion, there will be no infection'.[20] Although we know something about how *not* to compromise host resistance (by minimizing anoxia, shock, foreign bodies and dead tissue), we cannot as yet increase the defensive capabilities of our patients: this is a growing point of research.

Prophylactic antibiotics

Early attempts to prevent surgical wound infection by antibiotics were frustrated by the fact that they were given after the operation, often only when the patient had returned to the ward and the next 'drug round' was due. It was Burke's paper in 1961[21] that opened the door to successful random control clinical trials of antibiotic prophylaxis in gastro-intestinal surgery. He concluded that 'There is a definite short period when the developing staphylococcal dermal or incisional infection may be suppressed by antibiotics. This effective period begins the moment bacteria gain access to the tissue and is over in 3 hours. Systemic antibiotics have no effect on primary staphylococcal infections if the bacteria creating the infection have been in the tissue longer than 3 hours before the antibiotics are given. Antibiotics cause maximum suppression of infection if given before bacteria gain access to tissue.'

The first important clinical trial was by Polk and Lopez-Mayor.[22] They reported a reduction in wound infection rates in 68 gastroduodenal operations from 30.6 per cent in the control group to zero in the experimental group and from 30 per cent to 7.4 per cent in 104 colorectal operations. The experimental group were given cephaloridine 1 g immediately before, and 5 and 12 hours after, operation.

Since publication of this trial there has been a plethora of papers reporting clinical trials of various antibiotics for the prophylaxis of wound infection after abdominal operations. The principle that the antibiotic must be in the tissues at the time of contamination is firmly established. What are not so confidently known are the answers to the following questions.

- Which antibiotic or combination of antibiotics should be chosen?
- How many doses of antibiotic are needed?
- Should antibiotics be given systemically or locally or both?
- What is the place of pre-incisional intra-incisional injection of antibiotics?
- Is there a place for intra-operative peritoneal lavage with antiseptics or antibiotics?
- Have antiseptics any role in wound management?
- What special measures are necessary when pus is encountered in the abdomen?

Which antibiotic or combination of antibiotics should be chosen?

So many natural, semi-synthetic and synthetic antimicrobial agents are available that the choice must initially be made by reference to the following rules, bearing in mind that the final arbiter of effectiveness is the random control clinical trial of one agent against another:

1. The agent must have an *in vitro* spectrum of antibacterial action which includes all potential pathogens likely to be encountered in the operations undertaken. Infections associated with prosthetic implants are likely to be staphylococcal, whereas after upper gastro-intestinal operations they are likely to be by aerobic enterobacteria and after lower intestinal operations by aerobic together with anaerobic enterobacteria. There is a special danger of clostridial myonecrosis after lower limb amputations for gangrene, and the choice of antimicrobial prophylaxis must be made with this in mind.

2. The agent must be formulated in a parenteral (or rectal) presentation. In sick people about to undergo abdominal operations, oral administration of antibiotics is undesirable and unreliable.

3. The agent must be capable of diffusing into traumatized tissues in an active form. The ability of closely related antibiotics to do this varies widely; cephalothin, for example, is much less effective in this respect than cephaloridine.[23] It is the concentration in the *tissue*, not that in body fluids, that matters.

4. The agent must have no important toxic side-effects. In the cut and

thrust of commercial competition the toxic effects of antibiotics are likely to be exaggerated. Chloramphenicol is a rare cause of bone marrow suppression, cephaloridine – in combination with frusemide – of renal failure, latamoxef and other third generation cephalosporins of bleeding, and all penicillins of anaphylaxis.

5. The agent must have a reasonably long biologically active half-life within the body. The serum half-lives of some common antibiotics are given in Table 27.2.

Table 27.2 Serum half-lives of some penicillins and cephalosporins

Antibiotic	Half-life (hours)
Cephalothin	0.5
Piperacillin	0.5–1.2
Cefamandole	0.6
Cefoxitin	0.7
Cephradine	0.7
Ticarcillin	0.9
Cephaloridine	1.1
Cefuroxime	1.1
Ampicillin	1.3
Cefazolin	1.8
Ceftazidime	1.9
Latamoxef	2.2
Ceftriaxone	5.5–8.0

6. The agent chosen for prophylaxis should be one which is seldom used for therapy. Bacteria rapidly acquire resistance to antibiotics which are widely prescribed for treatment by virtue of plasmids which allow them to elaborate beta-lactamases and other resistance determinants. The antibiotics chosen for prophylaxis should either be relatively resistant to destruction by beta-lactamases (e.g. latamoxef) or be combined with clavulanic acid which destroys beta-lactamases (e.g. amoxycillin with clavulanic acid).

How many doses of antibiotic are needed?

I have already referred to Polk's important work which showed the benefit of a three-dose regimen.[22] Polk and Miles subsequently validated the concept of adding two postoperative doses to the pre-operative dose.[24] In mice injected intramuscularly with *E. coli* they found that the local defences reduced the bacterial population to 5 per cent within 4 hours, but that multiplication subsequently occurred and the bacteria were not finally eliminated until 72 hours after inoculation. The three-dose regimen was widely accepted, but clinical trials in my unit[25] and elsewhere failed to show additional benefit from postoperative antibiotics. Whether one chooses a single pre-operative dose, or whether one adds postoperative doses, there is no justification for continuing antibiotic prophylaxis beyond the day of operation. Antibiotics do not prevent ward-acquired infections, and their indiscriminate use for days or weeks can only result in acquisition of resistant and possibly more dangerous pathogens.

Should antibiotics be given systemically or locally or both?

The theoretical advantage of putting an antibiotic into the surgical wound is that a high local concentration is attained and that even relatively resistant organisms can be destroyed. A clinical trial of intravenous cephaloridine against intra-incisional cephaloridine, however, failed to substantiate this advantage.[26] It is common practice in many units to irrigate wounds with antibiotic solutions during operation, but whether this improves the wound infection rate over what is achieved by pre-operative parenteral antibiotic administration alone has not been established.

What is the place of pre-incisional intra-incisional injection of antibiotics?

This interesting concept was introduced by Taylor and his colleagues.[27] They injected 20 ml of a 5 per cent solution of cefoxitin into the subcutaneous tissues along the line of the proposed abdominal incision in 91 anaesthetized patients and compared the postoperative wound infection rate with that of 90 randomized controls given no antibiotic prophylaxis. Four of the 91 patients given cefoxitin developed wound infections in hospital, compared with 15 of the 90 controls. The method has the theoretical advantages of both intra-incisional and intravenous administration producing a high concentration of antibiotic at the site of potential parietal contamination and yet attaining reasonable blood levels. I am at present conducting a random control clinical trial of amoxycillin–clavulanic acid administered in this way against the same antibiotic injected intravenously at induction of anaesthesia.

Is there a place for intra-operative peritoneal and wound lavage with antibiotics or antiseptics?

Generations of surgeons trained in the Halsted tradition have gently irrigated surgical wounds with copious quantities of saline. This reduces the concentration of bacteria but is probably ineffective in reducing infection rates, and the addition of even relatively non-toxic antiseptics such as noxythiolin, polyvinylpyrrolidone-iodine or chlorhexidine almost certainly harms host defensive cells as much as bacteria.[28, 29, 30] For many years Matheson has used a 0.1 per cent solution of tetracycline for peritoneal and wound lavage, and an audit of 1504 consecutive operations disclosed a remarkably low rate of both intra-abdominal and wound infection, the latter being 3.5 per cent in clean operations, 1.5 per cent in clean-contaminated operations, 1.5 per cent in contaminated and 8.0 per cent in dirty operations.[31] A clinical trial in my unit, however, failed to achieve such excellent results with tetracycline lavage and showed significantly lower rates of wound infection in patients given a single pre-operative intravenous dose of 1 g of latamoxef.[32]

Have antiseptics any role in wound management?

Sixty years ago Fleming showed that all antiseptics then available were more toxic to neutrophils than to bacteria.[33] This important work profoundly influenced the direction of thought in the Department of Microbiology at St. Mary's Hospital in London towards methods of stimulating the immune system. Under the direction of Sir Almroth Wright, the department was named the Inoculation Department. So convinced was Wright that no good would come out of a search for chemicals with a selective action against bacteria that Fleming received little support for the purification of penicillin, and it was not until over a decade after its discovery that Florey and Chain succeeded in the task.

At the same time that Fleming published his work on antiseptics, Moynihan wrote that 'Every operation in surgery is an experiment in bacteriology. . . . Our bacteriological experiment may be conducted with one of two intentions: (1) The exclusion of all organisms from the wound: (2) The destruction of all organisms reaching the wound, by a bactericide applied to the wound surfaces'.[34] The attraction of chemical rather than antibiotic prophylaxis is that bacteria do not acquire resistance to antiseptics as readily as they do to antibiotics, and the introduction of relatively non-toxic antiseptics stimulated a burst of enquiry into their role in the prevention of wound infection. The antiseptic most favoured has been povidone iodine. It is rapidly bactericidal and has less toxicity against host cells than traditional antiseptics. Gilmore found that the application of povidone iodine powder to abdominal surgical wounds significantly reduced the wound infection rate compared with untreated controls.[35] Work in my unit, however, showed that it is inferior to cephaloridine for this purpose.[36]

What special measures are necessary when pus is encountered in the abdomen?

Abdominal surgical incisions for the treatment of septic peritonitis or abscess are singularly liable to become infected, and the infection may be so severe as to cause digestion of the abdominal wall and dehiscence of the wound. It is in these circumstances that the practice of non-closure (or delayed closure) of the wound is so valuable.[37] Usually, the omission of skin closure is all that is necessary, but there are two conditions in which avoidance of aponeurotic sutures is also indicated: when stercoral or traumatic perforation of the colon has allowed the escape of faeces into the peritoneal cavity, and when the operation is undertaken for a complex pancreatic abscess. In both cases the technique of non-closure allows two benefits: reduction in dangerous wound infection, and easy re-exploration for residual intra-abdominal sepsis. The escape of abdominal viscera is prevented by a gauze dressing, which is changed daily under general anaesthesia and further pockets of pus evacuated.

I have recently been attracted to the use of strings of polymethylmethacrylate beads incorporating gentamicin (Septopal) as an alternative to non-closure of these grossly contaminated surgical wounds. These are left in the subcutaneous tissue for 5 days and then removed; my preliminary observations are favourable. A controlled clinical trial of the two methods is still in progress.

Conclusion

Primary surgical wound infection is caused by bacterial contamination of the wound during operation. In abdominal operations the source of these bacteria is mainly endogenous, and prophylaxis requires emptying and – if possible – sterilizing viscera which are to be incised or excised, the avoidance of parietal contamination and the use of appropriate antibiotics before, or during, the operation. Grossly contaminated surgical wounds should not be closed primarily.

References

1. Burn JI, Sellwood RA, Okubadejo OA, Welbourn RB. Preoperative bowel sterilization. *Postgrad Med J* 1967; **43**:17–21.
2. Bartlett JG, Condon RE, Gorbach SL, Clarke JS, Nichols RL, Ochi S. Veterans Administration cooperative study on bowel preparation for elective colorectal operations: impact of oral antibiotic regimen on colonic flora, wound irrigation cultures and bacteriology of septic complications. *Ann Surg* 1978; **188**:249–54.
3. Stone HH, Hooper CA, Kolb LD, Geheber CE, Dawkins EJ. Antibiotic prophylaxis in gastric, biliary and colonic surgery. *Ann Surg* 1976; **184**: 443–52.
4. Pollock AV, Evans M, Parida S. The prediction of abdominal surgical wound infection: the value of an enrichment broth for initial culture of operative parietal swabs. *J Hosp Infect* 1986; **8**: 242–47.
5. Radcliffe AG, Dudley HAF. Intra-operative antegrade irrigation of the large intestine. *Surg Gynec Obstet* 1983; **156**:721–23.
6. Jones FE, DeCosse JJ, Condon RE. Evaluation of 'instant' preparation of the colon with povidone iodine. *Ann Surg* 1976; **184**:74–79.
7. Garlock JH, Seley GP. The use of sulfanilamide in surgery of the colon and rectum. Preliminary report. *Surgery* 1939; **5**:787–90.
8. Poth EJ. Historical development of intestinal antisepsis. *World J Surg* 1982; **6**: 153–59.
9. Rosenberg IL, Graham NG, de Dombal FT, Goligher JC. Preparation of the intestine in patients undergoing major large-bowel surgery, mainly for neoplasms of the colon and rectum. *Brit J Surg* 1971; **58**:266–69.
10. Washington JA II, Dearing WH, Judd ES, Elveback LR. Effect of pre-operative antibiotic regimen on development of infection after intestinal surgery. *Ann Surg* 1974; **180**:567–72.
11. Clarke JS, Condon RE, Bartlett JG, Gorbach SL, Nichols RL, Ochi S. Pre-operative oral antibiotics reduce septic complications of colon operations. Results of a prospective randomized double-blind study. *Ann Surg* 1977; **186**:251–59.
12. Tally FP, Sutter VL, Finegold SM. Metronidazole versus anaerobes. *In vitro* data and initial clinical observations. *Calif Med* 1972; **117**:22–26.
13. Goldring J, Scott A, McNaught W, Gillespie G. Prophylactic oral antimicrobial agents in elective colonic surgery. A controlled trial. *Lancet* 1975; **ii**:997–1000.
14. Pollock AV, Evans M. Antimicrobial preparation of the colon. *New Eng J Med* 1980; **303**:1066.
15. Cole WR, Bernard HR. Wound isolation in the prevention of postoperative wound infection. *Surg Gynec Obstet* 1967; **125**:257–60.
16. Alexander Williams J, Oates GD, Brown PP *et al*. Abdominal wound infections and plastic wound guards. *Brit J Surg* 1972; **59**:142–46.
17. Psaila JV, Wheeler MH, Crosby DL. The role of plastic wound drapes in the prevention of wound infection following abdominal surgery. *Brit J Surg* 1977; **64**:729–32.

18. Pollock AV. Prevention of wound infection by an antiseptic wound protector. *J Roy Soc Med* 1980; **73**:831.
19. Pollock AV. The present position of prophylaxis in surgical sepsis. In: Taylor I. (ed) *Progress in Surgery, Volume I*. Churchill Livingstone, Edinburgh, 1985, pp 10–25.
20. Burke JF. Ashley A. Miles and the prevention of infection following surgery. *Arch Surg* 1984; **119**:17–19.
21. Burke JF. The effective period of preventive antibiotic action in experimental incisions and dermal lesions. *Surgery* 1961; **50**:161–68.
22. Polk HC Jr, Lopez-Mayor JF. Postoperative wound infection: a prospective study of determinant factors and prevention. *Surgery* 1969; **66**:97–103.
23. Polk HC Jr, In: Discussion of Burdon JGW, Morris PJ, Hunt P, Watts JMcK. A trial of cephalothin sodium in colon surgery to prevent wound infection. *Arch Surg* 1977; **112**:1169–73.
24. Polk HC Jr, Miles AA. The decisive period in the primary infection of muscle by *Escherichia coli. Brit J Exper Path* 1973; **54**:99–109.
25. Brennan SS, Pickford IR, Evans M, Pollock AV. The prophylaxis of wound infection after abdominal operations: is one dose of antibiotic enough? *J Hosp Infect* 1982; **3**:351–56.
26. Greenall MJ, Atkinson JE, Evans M, Pollock AV. Single-dose antibiotic prophylaxis of surgical wound sepsis: which route of administration is best? A controlled trial of intra-incisional and intravenous cephaloridine. *J Antimicrob Chemother* 1981; **7**:223–27.
27. Taylor TV, Walker WS, Mason RC, Richmond J, Lee D. Pre-operative intra-parietal (intra-incisional) cefoxitin in abdominal surgery. *Brit J Surg* 1982; **69**:461–62.
28. Pollock AV, Froome K, Evans M. The bacteriology of primary wound sepsis in potentially contaminated abdominal operations: the effect of irrigation, povidone iodine and cephaloridine on the sepsis rate assessed in a clinical trial. *Brit J Surg* 1978; **65**:76–80.
29. Kuijpers HC. Is prophylactic abdominal irrigation with polyvinylpyrrolidone iodine (PVPI) safe? *Dis Col Rect* 1985; **28**:481–83.
30. Brennan SS, Leaper DJ. The effect of antiseptics on the healing wound: a study using the rabbit ear chamber. *Brit J Surg* 1985; **72**:780–82.
31. Krukowski ZH, Stewart MPM, Alsayer HM, Matheson NA. Infection after abdominal surgery: five year prospective study. *Brit Med J* 1984; **288**:278–80.
32. Sauven P, Playforth MJ, Smith GMR, Evans M, Pollock AV. Single dose antibiotic prophylaxis of abdominal surgical wound infection: a trial of pre-operative latamoxef against peroperative tetracycline lavage. *J Roy Soc Med* 1986; **79**:137–141.
33. Fleming A. The action of chemical and physiological antiseptics in a septic wound. *Brit J Surg* 1919–20; **7**:99–129.
34. Moynihan BGA. The ritual of a surgical operation. *Brit J Surg* 1920; **8**:27–35.
35. Gilmore OJA. A reappraisal of the use of antiseptics in surgical practice. *Ann Roy Coll Surg Engl* 1977; **59**:93–103.
36. Pollock AV, Evans M. Povidone iodine for the control of surgical wound infection: a controlled clinical trial against cephaloridine. *Brit J Surg* 1975; **62**:292–94.
37. Brennan SS, Smith GMR, Evans M, Pollock AV. The management of the perforated appendix: a controlled clinical trial. *Brit J Surg* 1982; **69**:510–12.

28

Principles of pathogenesis and prevention of exogenous ward-acquired infections

The concentration of sick people into a single building has a long and admirable history, but it is only in the last century that advances have been made in the prevention of hospital infections. Florence Nightingale, knowing nothing of bacteria, was horrified by the filth of the hospital at Scutari and later wrote that 'the very first requirement in a Hospital [is] that it should do the sick no harm'.

Since that time hospitals have become cleaner places, but patients are still at risk of acquiring infections while they are in hospital. How do these infections occur and how can they be prevented?

Role of attendants' hands

The resident bacterial flora of the skin is relatively harmless, but the hands of nurses and doctors are easily contaminated by transient pathogens which can then be passed from patient to patient. These transient pathogens are easily washed off by soap and water, or more effectively by an antiseptic detergent solution – chlorhexidine or povidone iodine. The advantage of the antiseptic wash is that it remains bactericidal for some hours. A 70 per cent alcohol or chlorhexidine-in-alcohol rinse results in even better eradication of skin bacteria when the hands are socially clean.

In circumstances in which exogenous infection is common and life-threatening, for example in intensive care units, it is customary to issue standing orders that attendants shall wash their hands or rinse them in alcoholic chlorhexidine after touching any patient. Broughall and his colleagues devised a monitoring system to record the frequency of hand-washing in a general ward and found that on average such nurse washed only 5–10 times during each shift,[1] which was far less than the estimated frequency. Unless the hands are contaminated with patients' secretions, it is preferable to instruct nurses to rinse in an alcoholic antiseptic after each patient contact. This is less likely to cause dermatitis – many people react unfavourably to repeated exposure to detergents.

Role of aerial cross infection

The design of hospital wards is still controversial. On the one hand, the 30- or 40-bed ward with beds against each long wall (the so-called Nightingale ward) is economical of nurses' time and allows continuous observation of all the patients. On the other hand, it is noisy, offends against personal privacy and allows airborne bacterial contamination from one patient to another. The alternatives are either all single rooms, or a mixture of single and four-bedded rooms. Twenty years ago a new hospital was built in Aberdeen and each room was plenum-ventilated. Smylie and his colleagues monitored the incidence of ward-acquired (secondary) wound infection by multi-resistant 'hospital' staphylococci and reported a 72 per cent reduction from that previously experienced in a Nightingale ward.[2]

We tend nowadays, however, to play down the role of airborne contamination in the aetiology of most nosocomial infections and concentrate attention on contamination of attendants' hands and of fluids which come into contact with patients. Maki and his colleagues cultured environmental swabs after commissioning a new hospital.[3] They found a significant increase in total positive cultures of the inanimate environment after 6–12 months of occupancy, but no more nosocomial infections than in the old hospital.

The part played by bacterial contamination of bed clothes, walls, floors and curtains in the aetiology of hospital-acquired infections is equally controversial, and most authorities decry routine environmental culturing and disinfection.[4]

Patients whose defences are grossly compromised, for example those who are neutropenic as a result of cytotoxic treatment, need to be treated using the most scrupulous aseptic techniques if they are to escape exogenous bacterial infection. So-called 'barrier' nursing techniques are inadequate for the protection of these patients, and there is some evidence that isolation in a clean air enclosure with 30–100 air changes per hour and a HEPA filter reduces the incidence of infections.[5] Whether this is a result of the clean air or whether it reminds attendants to wash their hands before attending to the patient remains conjectural.

Role of contaminated fluids

Bacterial contamination of commercially available intravenous solutions is rare, but the careless addition of other substances into a bag or bottle of intravenous fluid may allow access of microorganisms. Such additions must be carried out with the utmost aseptic precautions. Bacterial contamination (often by *Pseudomonas* species) of fluids such as mouth washes and the water in nebulizers is much more common.

Role of host defences

Sick people have less resistance to infection, and even light contamination by relatively harmless organisms, for example coagulase-negative staphylococci, can result in serious infection in patients in surgical intensive care units.[6] The importance of host defences against infection cannot be overemphasized.

Role of antibiotic abuse

Valuable as they are, antibiotics can be so over-prescribed that the hospital environment becomes contaminated by resistant organisms. Price and Sleigh were able to control an epidemic of *Klebsiella aerogenes* meningitis in a neurosurgical unit only after withdrawal of all antibiotics.[7] The prescription, particularly of broad-spectrum antibiotics, without microbiological justification and without removal of infected foci and drainage of abscesses can produce nothing but ill effects.

Control of ward-acquired infections

The most important person in the infection control team is the surveillance officer, usually a nurse. This person works in close collaboration with clinicans and microbiologists and should be in a position to bring to light undesirable practices and epidemic nosocomial infections. The job is facilitated if the Department of Microbiology records infections in their computer, not only by the names of patients, but also by the species of bacteria isolated. An outbreak of infection in any part of the hospital should alert clinicians immediately to the necessity for tightening up rules of asepsis in that department. I will discuss these rules in relation to specific infections in later chapters.

References

1. Broughall JM, Marshman C, Jackson B, Bird P. An automatic monitoring system for measuring handwashing frequency in hospital wards. *J Hosp Infect* 1984; **5**:447–53.
2. Smylie HG, Davidson AIG, Macdonald A, Smith G. Ward design in relation to postoperative wound infection: Part I. *Br Med J* 1971; **1**:67–72.
3. Maki DG, Alvarado GJ, Hassemer CA, Zilz MA. Relation of the inanimate hospital environment to endemic nosocomial infection. *New Engl J Med* 1982; **307**:1562–66.
4. Daschner FD. The cost of hospital-acquired infection. *J Hosp Infect* 1984; **5 (Suppl A)**:27–33.
5. Minns RJ, Cartner R. A portable clean air enclosure for neutropenic patients requiring hospital treatment: a preliminary study. *J Hosp Infect* 1983; **4**:406–409.
6. Meakins JL (ed). *Surgical Infection in Critical Care Medicine.* Edinburgh, Churchill Livingstone, 1985.
7. Price DJE, Sleigh JD. Control of infection due to *Klebsiella aerogenes* in a neuro-surgical unit by withdrawal of all antibiotics. *Lancet* 1970; **ii**:1213–15.

29

Secondary wound infection and wound dressings

An uncontaminated wound closed by sutures, tapes, clips or staples is immune to exogenous bacterial contamination within a few hours. Experimental guinea-pig wounds closed by tapes were more resistant to infection after surface contamination by *Staphylococcus aureus* or *Escherichia coli* than sutured wounds, and large numbers of bacteria (10^9) were required to cause wound infections.[1] Two hours after wound closure by tapes no infection was caused by either organism, whereas sutured wounds were more vulnerable, surface contamination after 2 hours with *E. coli* resulting in 57 per cent infections and contamination with *Staph. aureus* resulting in 10 per cent infections.

From the clinical standpoint, these results confirm the acceptance that a closed surgical wound does not become infected after the patient has been returned from the operating theatre as long as it remains dry. Quite different considerations, however, govern the behaviour of wet wounds, whether they are wet because they lack skin cover or whether the fluid discharges from the sutured wound for some other reason. Such a wound is susceptible to ward-acquired exogenous infection either from the patient's own microflora, from the hands of attendants or occasionally from the air. It is for these wounds that surgical dressings are important.

Requirements of a surgical dressing

- The surgical dressing must be sterile. A working party of the British Public Health Laboratory Service and the Division of Hospital Infection at the Central Public Health Laboratory investigated the sterility of packaged dressings of British and Indian manufacture.[2] They found evidence of failure of sterilization and of later contamination during the manufacture of many dressings originating from India. The level of contamination was low, and the bacteria isolated were of low pathogenicity, but even such contamination is unacceptable.
- The dressing must absorb secretions without desiccating the healing wound. The ingrowth of fragile epithelium is inhibited by dryness.[3] Traditional cotton-based dressings can result in desiccation of open wounds.
- The dressing must prevent access to the wound by exogenous micro-organisms.
- The dressing must not shed fibres which can act as foreign bodies, potentiating infection and delaying healing.

- Replacement of the dressing must be effected without causing pain and damaging the healing process. Gauze dressings absorb plasma which then clots and dries and may cause adherence to the surface of the wound.
- The dressing must not liberate harmful chemicals, including antiseptics. Sixty years ago Fleming concluded that all antiseptics are more harmful to leucocytes than to bacteria,[4] and recent work with a rabbit ear chamber model using the less toxic antiseptics – povidone-iodine and chlorhexidine – showed that they also interfered with healing.[5]
- Different considerations govern the requirements of dressings for wounds which are already infected. Here the problem is not only to prevent superinfection but also to remove sloughs and other debris and expose healthy granulation tissue over which epithelium can grow.

Choice of wound dressing

Cotton-based dressings

Layers of gauze are more absorbent than any other dressing and are more widely used. Closed wounds need only three or four layers of sterile gauze attached by adhesive tape or bandages. For the first-aid management of open traumatic wounds a thicker, cotton-based dressing is appropriate – for example, a field dressing. Such dressings are also appropriate for the postoperative management of surgical wounds which have been deliberately left unsutured – for example, after anal surgery, incision of an abscess or laparotomy for faecal peritonitis.

Non-adherent gauze

Gauze with one face covered by polyurethane film does not stick to the wound but is less absorbent than plain gauze. Paraffin-covered open weave gauze (tulle gras) is useful for covering the recipient site of skin grafts. It must be backed by absorbent cotton dressings.

Semi-permeable adhesive films

Adhesive transparent polyurethane films, such as 'Opsite', have transformed the management of the donor site after split skin grafting. They are comfortable, allow transpiration of water vapour and oxygen, and do not need to be removed until the wound has healed. For other wounds their place is less well-defined, but they may be valuable for covering partial-thickness burns.[6] Their drawback is that they do not allow the egress of fluid, which can collect under the film and strip it away from the surrounding skin. Frequent aspiration of this fluid must be carried out with strict attention to asepsis so as to avoid exogenous bacterial contamination.

Hydrogel dressings

Polyacrylamide flexible transparent dressings conform to the contours of a wound and are non-adherent and comfortable. They are capable of preventing ingress of microorganisms, but those already present in the wound, particularly *Pseudomonas aeruginosa*, can multiply and delay healing.[7]

Silicone foam elastomer

This product of Dow Corning forms a flexible mould in a deep wound and is comfortable. Its use is primarily to prevent premature skin healing in deep wounds, for example after excision of pilonidal sinuses. It does not absorb secretions but can be washed and replaced by the patient, resulting in considerable saving of nursing time.

Dressings for infected wounds

The aim in this case is not only to prevent exogenous superinfection, but also to encourage the removal of dead tissue. Numerous chemicals which either remove sloughs mechanically, like hydrogen peroxide, or digest them (e.g. papain) have been advocated. They are all toxic to leucocytes, and their beneficial effects are probably related more to the frequent wet dressings which are necessary than to any chemical actions. My own preference is for plain sterile saline-soaked gauze covered with a polyethylene bandage. Infected wounds and ulcers on the extremities can conveniently be managed by enclosing the limb in a polyethylene bag and irrigating with saline. On the trunk an infected wound can conveniently be irrigated through an adherent domed plastic cup (Squibb Wound Irrigation Device).

Dry porous hydrophilic beads ('Debrisan') may be useful in debridement of discharging infected wounds covered by slough.[8] They depend for their action on maintaining the wetness of the wound and need frequent replacement after irrigating away the spent beads. They are expensive not only in themselves but also in terms of nursing time.

Summary

Wounds which are covered by skin and remain dry during the healing process are immune to exogenous ward-acquired infection. Wet wounds are vulnerable and must be protected from bacterial contamination by observance of aseptic rituals and by the use of sterile dressings. The most generally useful dressings are cotton-based, but there are occasions when some of the newer synthetic dressings are better.

References

1. Schauerhamer RA, Edlich RF, Panek P, Thul J, Prusak M, Wangensteen OH. Studies in the management of the contaminated wound. VII Susceptibility of surgical wounds to postoperative surface contamination. *Am J Surg* 1971; **122**:74–77.

2. Marples RR. Contaminated first-aid dressings: report of a working party of the PHLS. *J Hygeine (Camb)* 1983; **90**:241–52.
3. Lawrence JC. What material for dressings? *Injury* 1982; **13**:500–512.
4. Fleming A. The action of chemical and physiological antiseptics in a septic wound. *Br J Surg* 1919–20; **7**:99–129.
5. Brennan SS, Leaper DJ. The effect of antiseptics on the healing wound: a study using the rabbit ear chamber. *Br J Surg* 1985; **72**:780–782.
6. Davies JWL. Synthetic materials for covering burn wounds: progress towards perfection. I Short-term dressing materials. *Burns* 1983; **10**:94–103.
7. Leaper DJ, Brennan SS, Simpson RA, Foster ME. Experimental infection and hydrogel dressings. *J Hosp Infect* 1985; **5 (suppl A)**:69–73.
8. Mummery RV, Richardson WW. Clinical trial of Debrisan in superficial ulceration. *J Internat Med Res* 1979; **7**:263–71.

30

Exogenous urinary tract infections

The distal urethra in both men and women is commonly colonized by intestinal and skin bacteria. These do not normally penetrate into the proximal urethra and bladder, but the presence of a urethral catheter can allow endogenous or exogenous bacteria access to the bladder. There are two opinions about the route of ascent of bacteria – either between the catheter and the urethral wall, or along the lumen of the catheter.[1] There is no evidence that application of antiseptics to the catheter-meatus junction is of value, but there is no doubt that closed drainage of the catheter into a sterile bag or bottle is preferable to open drainage or the use of a spigot.

Exogenous infection can, however, occur if the catheter-bag connection is taken down, as it may have to be to evacuate clots, or if the bag is emptied carelessly and without strict asepsis. In a prospective study Blenkharn found that 137 of 512 catheterized patients (27 per cent) in an intensive care unit developed urinary infections despite the use of a closed system of drainage.[2] 'Resident' ward organisms, *Pseudomonas aeruginosa* and *Klebsiella aerogenes* accounted for 52 (38 per cent) and 28 (20 per cent) infections respectively. He showed that the incidence of acquired infection was halved in a subsequent series of 576 patients after the introduction of a new closed system ('Ureofix 500'). *Ps. aeruginosa* and *K. aerogenes* were cultured from urine in only 3 (4 per cent) and 4 (6 per cent) of the 70 infected patients in the second series.

The incidence of catheter-associated urinary tract infection can be reduced by observance of the following rules:

- Avoid catheterization if possible. If the catheter is inserted merely to sample the urine for biochemical or microbiological tests, substitute a regimen of 'clean catch' urine sampling or aspirate urine from the bladder by suprapubic puncture.
- If catheterization is essential because of postoperative urine retention, it is safer to introduce a fine-bore catheter, drain the urine and remove the catheter. Workers in Leiden conducted a random control trial in orthopaedic patients requiring intermittent urethral catheterization.[3] They showed a reduction in the incidence of nosocomial urinary tract infections from 28 per cent to 4 per cent by instilling 50 ml of 2 per cent povidone iodine into the bladder after draining the urine.
- In any case, introduce the catheter – without touching its surface – after cleansing the meatus with chlorhexidine or povidone iodine

detergent. Connect the catheter immediately to sterile tubing leading
to a sterile bag.

- If the catheter is to be left in place, empty the bag without contaminating the port.
- Remove the catheter as soon as possible. Ideally, the catheter should remain in place for less than 3 days, after which each additional day brings additional danger of infection.

There are many variations on these rules, most of which have not been proved to be effective. These variations include the use of antiseptic or antibiotic lubricants during catheterization, the addition of antiseptics to the drainage bag, the use of antiseptic bladder irrigations and of prophylactic systemic antibacterial drugs – all these are of doubtful value. Systemic antibacterials, whether they be antibiotics, sulphonamides, trimethoprim, nitrofurantoin, nalidixic acid or the newer quinolones such as ciprofloxacin, should be used only to treat, not to prevent, urinary tract infections, and then preferably after removal of the catheter.

Urinary tract infections in patients with spinal injuries[4]

The immediate result of a spinal cord lesion is spinal shock – total paralysis below the site of the lesion. This condition lasts some weeks and is succeeded either by partial recovery of voluntary movement or by spinal reflex activity. The bladder, previously a flaccid bag, now responds to suprapubic percussion by contracting, and its emptying can be further improved by suprapubic pressure. Vesico-ureteric incompetence leads to dilatation of the upper urinary tract and infection of the bladder can then result in pyelonephritis. Urea-splitting organisms, particularly *Proteus* species, cause the urine to become alkaline and thus facilitate stone formation in the bladder and kidneys.

The initial management of a paralysed bladder is best accomplished by 6-hourly catheterization, using a fine-bore (12 or 14 FG) catheter. An indwelling urethral or suprapubic catheter inevitably results in infection. After a few weeks (during which time the urine is examined microbiologically at least once a week and any infection treated by an appropriate antimicrobial agent) it may be possible to get the bladder to empty by intermittent suprapubic percussion and expression. Failing this, intermittent self-catheterization is preferable to an indwelling catheter and, particularly in women who are incontinent in spite of percussion and expression, intermittent self-catheterization is proper treatment. In elderly, frail people, and in those with reduced hand movements, an indwelling catheter may be inevitable. In these cases infection is inevitable, and the patient is best served by drugs such as ascorbic acid which acidify the urine and prevent stone formation.

References

1. Gillespie WA, Simpson RA, Jones JE, Nashef L, Teasdale C, Speller DC. Does the addition of disinfectant to urine drainage bags prevent infection in catheterized patients? *Lancet* 1983; 1:1037–39.

2. Blenkharn JJ. Prevention of bacteriuria during urinary catheterization of patients in an intensive care unit: evaluation of the 'Ureofix 500' closed drainage system. *J Hosp Infect* 1985; **6**:187–93.
3. van den Brock PJ, Daha TJ, Mouton RP. Bladder irrigation with povidone iodine in prevention of urinary tract infections associated with intermittent urethral catheterization. *Lancet* 1985; **i**:563–65.
4. Grundy D, Russell J. Urological management of spinal cord injury. *Br Med J* 1986; **292**:249–53.

31

Exogenous bronchopulmonary infections

I have considered the most lethal pulmonary complication of shock and sepsis – adult respiratory distress syndrome – in Chapter 6. The following discussion concerns postoperative hospital-acquired chest infections. The incidence of these infections after operations which do not include incisions in the chest or abdomen is negligible.[1] After abdominal operations, however, they rank with postoperative wound infections as important causes of illness and, occasionally, death. Most of these infections are of exogenous origin, but it is impossible in many cases to discern whether the bacterial contamination has taken place in the operating theatre or in the ward. Endogenous bronchopulmonary enteric bacterial contamination can, however, occur. The organisms are usually Gram-negative, and infection follows inhalation of contaminated gastric contents by patients with postoperative ileus and those in intensive care units treated with antacids or cimetidine.[2]

In a consecutive series of 1207 elective and emergency major laparotomies I found that enteric organisms were cultured from sputum postoperatively in 85 patients (7 per cent). The presence of a nasogastric tube increased the chances of this happening: Gram-negative rods were recovered from the sputum in 11 per cent of 535 patients who had a tube and in 4 per cent of 653 patients who did not. In a random control clinical trial Cheadle and his colleagues found that the combination of nasogastric intubation and cimetidine resulted in a significantly higher incidence of postoperative pneumonia.[3]

It is quite common for potential respiratory pathogens, particularly *Streptococcus pneumoniae* and *Haemophilus influenzae* to live harmlessly in the pharynx. Tebbutt reported the recovery of the *H. influenzae* from throat swabs of 28 of 192 patients (14.6 per cent) admitted to hospital for elective surgical operations.[4] In only three of these (two of whom were chronic bronchitics) did a *Haemophilus* chest infection follow operation.

Causes of postoperative pulmonary infections

The essential cause of these infections is bacterial contamination of the bronchi, bronchioles and alveoli following an incision in the chest or abdomen; the pain from the incision inhibits coughing, deep breathing and periodic sighing, thus allowing lobular collapse and accumulation of sputum. General anaesthesia *per se* probably plays only a small part, patients who have had operations under local or regional anaesthesia being just as prone to chest complications.[5] General anaesthesia involving the passage of an endotracheal tube may, however, allow bacterial colonization of the bronchi which, in the absence of efficient clearing of secretions by forced expiratory efforts and by ciliary action, can allow the development of infection and invasion of bacteria into pulmonary parenchyma.

Sex, smoking and bronchitis

In the consecutive series of 1207 major laparotomies mentioned above, I recorded postoperative chest complications by scoring their most serious manifestation. The score is as follows:[6]

Score	Sign or symptom
1	New or increased cough
1	New or increased sputum
1	Clinical or radiographic signs in the chest
3	Pyrexia 38°C or more for 48 hours or more associated with pulmonary signs and symptoms
3	Purulent sputum or pathogens cultured from sputum
5	Therapeutic bronchoscopy, tracheostomy, or endotracheal intubation

If the postoperative chest score was 0–3, I regarded the patient as free of significant pulmonary complications, whereas I regarded a score of 4 or more as clinically significant. Using this scoring system I found that men who smoked or who had pre-existing chronic bronchitis were more likely to have significant chest complications than those who were non-smokers or who did not suffer from chronic bronchitis. The incidence was 157 out of 393 (40 per cent) in the former and 43 out of 174 (25 per cent) in the latter. Women, whether or not they smoked or had chronic bronchitis, fared better than men, the smokers or bronchitics having an incidence of significant postoperative chest infection of 62 out of 302 (21 per cent) compared with their healthier sisters, 30 of whom out of 319 (9 per cent) suffered chest infections.

Depressed ventilation

All major laparotomies result in depression of ventilation, whether this is measured by peak expiratory flow rate, forced expiratory volume in 1 second, forced vital capacity or arterial oxygen tension. The amount of depression correlates well with the amount of pain from the incision but weakly with the development of chest complications. Upper abdominal incisions cause more depression than lower, and long incisions cause more depression than short. I have not found any alteration in laparotomy technique (transverse or vertical incisions, or method or material for suturing the musculoaponeurosis) which has any bearing on postoperative ventilatory function or the development of chest complications.

Micro-embolization

One of the main effects of postoperative pulmonary dysfunction is a reduction in arterial oxygen tension which may persist for up to 1 week and is exacerbated if pulmonary infection occurs. The reduction in P_aO_2 is the result of either venous blood in pulmonary arterioles flowing through capillaries in the walls of alveoli which are airless, or the shunting of venous blood through arteriovenous channels so that it does not come into proximity with air. The importance of the latter mechanism has been stressed by the finding of platelet aggregates in venous blood after operations. McCollum and Campbell tested the venous blood filtration pressure through a Swank screen filter without the addition of anticoagulants, and they showed that this pressure correlated with the presence of platelet aggregates seen on the filter by scanning electron micrography.[7] In 20 patients they found that the higher the screen filtration pressure, the lower the arterial oxygen tension, on postoperative days 1 and 7. They concluded that platelet aggregates blocked terminal pulmonary arterioles and led to the opening up of arteriovenous channels.

Embolization of major pulmonary arteries is rare, and has become more rare since the widespread use of prophylactic subcutaneous low-dose heparin. It results in pulmonary insufficiency, but death as a result of major pulmonary embolism is cardiac, not pulmonary.

Prolonged endotracheal intubation

There is little doubt that the treatment of respiratory failure by endotracheal intubation with intermittent positive pressure ventilation prevents death in some patients who 'seemed to be spending more effort breathing than they could keep up'.[8] Endotracheal tubes, however, may allow bacterial colonization of the upper airways, with subsequent invasion of bronchi and lungs. The longer a patient stays in a respiratory intensive care unit, the more likely he or she is to develop nosocomial pulmonary infection – 96 per cent of patients who stayed more than 1 week in an intensive care unit in Glasgow developed infection.[9]

Johanson and his colleagues found that pharyngeal colonization by Gram-negative aerobes, particularly *Pseudomonas aeruginosa*, *Klebsiella* spp., *Escherichia coli* and *Proteus* spp. was common in seriously ill patients,[10] especially when they had endotracheal tubes or prolonged antibacterial treatment. Pneumonia occurred in 23 per cent of these patients, compared with 3.3 per cent of those in whom colonization was not detected.

Prophylaxis of bronchopulmonary infection

The rules are few, and sometimes impossible to reconcile with other aspects of patient care. They are:

- prevent bacterial colonization of the respiratory tract
- prevent pulmonary atelectasis which encourages infection
- use antibiotics circumspectly

Prevention of bacterial colonization of the respiratory tract

Avoidance of nasogastric tubes

There is sound evidence that the presence of a nasogastric tube predisposes to bronchial bacterial colonization and that the longer the tube remains in place, the greater the risk. Argov and his colleagues used nasogastric decompression after 150 consecutive upper abdominal operations, and in the next 150 operations did not use a tube.[11] In the first 150 patients there were 23 who developed pneumonia, compared with 2 in the group of patients without a tube. When gastric decompression is essential, it is preferable to insert a gastrostomy tube.

Maintenance of sterility of respiratory care equipment

Some Gram-negative rods, notably *Ps. aeruginosa* and *Legionella pneumophila*, are capable of multiplying in apparently nutrient-free aqueous solutions including tap water. It is important, therefore, that the water in humidifiers and nebulizers be sterile and that humidifiers be maintained at a bacteriostatic temperature of 60°C and that nebulizers be sterilized daily.[12]

All parts of anaesthetic and respiratory support equipment can become contaminated by bacteria, and it is impracticable to sterilize them in an autoclave. Ethylene oxide gas cannot be used because it is toxic to tissues and is absorbed and slowly released over several days by rubber and plastic. Thorough detergent cleansing followed by immersion in 2 per cent buffered glutaraldehyde for 30 minutes, followed by washing in sterile water, is probably adequate for all equipment except tracheostomy tubes which must be sterilized or disposable. Respirators are difficult to disinfect, but detachable autoclavable patient circuits are available and have been in routine use in Oslo for 10 years.[12]

Tracheal suction is essential for patients who are unable to cough up sputum. The suction apparatus must be autoclaved every day and used for only one patient at a time. Tracheal catheters must be sterile (usually disposable) and handled only with sterile gloves.

Prevention of pulmonary atelectasis

Alveoli are kept open because the pressure of air within them is greater than the (negative) intrapleural pressure. Postoperative atelectasis is associated not only with retention of bronchial secretions but with monotonous breathing uninterrupted by periodic sighing. Prophylaxis involves the encouragement of deep breathing, the use of the Bartlett Incentive Spirometer or the cheaper Uniflo and Triflo Respiratory Exercisers.[13] Repeated heavy chest percussion with postural drainage encourages the patient to expectorate secretions. In weak and uncooperative patients it may be necessary to remove tracheo-bronchial fluid by blind or bronchoscopic endotracheal catheterization, or percutaneous intratracheal injection of 5 ml of sterile saline.

Circumspect use of prophylactic antibiotics

There is little evidence that the routine prophylactic use of antibiotics has any effect on the incidence of hospital-acquired respiratory tract infections, and there is circumstantial evidence that prolonged courses of antibiotics favour the development of fungal and exotic bacterial infections. The scant evidence in favour of prophylactic antibiotics comes from two trials: Galland and his colleagues reported only five cases of pneumonia (15 per cent) after 33 cardiac operations in patients given three peri-operative doses of cefamandole, compared with a control group given cephradine for 3 days in whom 18 out of 42 (43 per cent) developed pneumonia.[14] In a trial of single-dose pre-operative intravenous cotrimoxazole for the prophylaxis of surgical wound infection after cholecystectomy, Morran and McArdle reported three chest infections (9 per cent) after 34 operations in the antibiotic group compared with 11 out of 34 (32 per cent) in the control group.[15]

My own experience is that none of the numerous antibiotics which I have tested in a series of random control trials of the prophylaxis of surgical wound infection has had any effect on the incidence of postoperative chest infections. As for antibiotic prophylaxis in respiratory intensive care units, more harm than good will result. Appropriate antibiotic treatment of established infection is, of course, an entirely different matter; it is essential, and there is some evidence that aerosol inhalation of antibiotics may be more effective than systemic treatment.[16]

Summary

Nosocomial bronchopulmonary infections are common after major abdominal and thoracic operations. They affect mainly men who smoke or who suffer from chronic bronchitis, those whose ventilatory function is reduced and those requiring prolonged endotracheal intubation. Prophylaxis must concentrate on the prevention of bacterial colonization of the respiratory tract and the prevention of pulmonary atelectasis. Antibiotics play an important part in treatment, but not in prophylaxis.

References

1. Garibaldi RTA, Britt MR, Coleman ML, Reading JC, Pace NL. Risk factors for postoperative pneumonia. *Am J Med* 1981; **70**:677–80.
2. Du Moulin GC, Hedley-Whyte J, Paterson DG, Lisbon A. Aspiration of gastric bacteria in antacid-treated patients: a frequent cause of postoperative colonization. *Lancet* 1982; **i**:242–45.
3. Cheadle WG, Vitale GC, Mackie CR. Prophylactic postoperative nasogastric decompression. A prospective study of its requirement and the influence of cimetidine in 200 patients. *Ann Surg.* 1985; **202**:361–66.
4. Tebbut GM. Study of postoperative chest infections with particular emphasis on those caused by *Haemophilus influenzae. J Clin Path* 1986; **39**:78–83.
5. Godfrey PJ, Greenan J, Ranasinghe DD, Shabestary SM, Pollock AV. Ventilatory capacity after three methods of anaesthesia for inguinal hernia repair: a randomized controlled trial. *Br J Surg* 1981; **68**:587–89.
6. Leaper DJ, Pollock AV, Evans M. Abdominal wound closure: a trial of nylon, polyglycolic acid and steel sutures. *Br J Surg* 1977; **64**:603–606.

7. McCollum CN, Campbell IT. The value of measuring platelet aggregates in the prediction of postoperative pulmonary dysfunction. *Br J Surg* 1979; **66**:703-707.
8. Peters RM, Hilberman M, Hogan JS, Crawford DA. Objective indications for respirator therapy in post-trauma and postoperative patients. *Am J Surg* 1972; **124**:262-69.
9. Thorp JM, Richards WC, Telfer ABM. A survey of infection in an intensive care unit. *Anaesthesia* 1979; **34**:643-49.
10. Johanson WG, Pierce AK, Sanford JP, Thomas GD. Nosocomial respiratory infection with Gram-negative bacilli. The significance of colonization of the respiratory tract. *Ann Intern Med* 1972; **77**:701-706.
11. Argov S, Goldstein I, Barzilai A. Is routine use of the nasogastric tube justified in upper abdominal surgery? *Am J Surg* 1980; **139**:849-50.
12. Hovig B. Lower respiratory tract infections associated with respiratory therapy and anaesthesia equipment. *J Hosp Infect* 1981; **2**:301-305.
13. Bartlett RH, Brennan ML, Gazzaniga AB, Hanson EL. Studies on the pathogenesis and prevention of postoperative pulmonary complications. *Surg Gynecol Obstet* 1973; **137**:925-33.
14. Galland RB, Shama Prenger KB, Darrell JH. Peroperative antibiotics in the prevention of chest infection following cardiac operations. *Br J Surg* 1980; **67**:97-98.
15. Morran C, McArdle CS. The reduction of postoperative chest infection by prophylactic co-trimoxazole. *Br J Surg* 1980; **67**:464-66.
16. Hodson ME, Penketh ARL, Batten JC. Aerosol carbenicillin and gentamicin treatment of *Pseudomonas aeruginosa* infection in patients with cystic fibrosis. *Lancet* 1981; **ii**:1137-39.

32

Infections caused by catheters, cannulae and other devices

Any tube which leads from contaminated skin to sterile organs or tissues is liable to introduce infection, but infections may occasionally also complicate the use of totally implanted devices such as ventriculo-peritoneal and peritoneo-venous shunts and pacemakers. I discuss infections of prosthetic arteries and joints in Chapter 25.

Urinary catheters

Hospital-acquired urinary tract infection is common (Fig. 32.1). Catheters are used not only in patients unable to pass urine, but also for monitoring urine output in the seriously ill. The incidence of bacteriuria following catheterization is closely related to the duration of catheterization, but can be reduced by adoption of strictly aseptic closed drainage systems.[1] There is some evidence that suprapubic cystostomy carries a lower risk of infection than urethral catheterization, and that intermittent passage of a catheter is less likely to result in infection than the use of an indwelling catheter.

There have been numerous attempts to reduce the incidence of catheter-associated bacteriuria by application of antiseptics around the external meatus, by the use of catheters impregnated with antiseptics, and by the

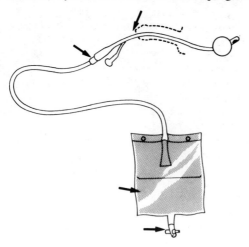

Fig. 32.1 Routes of infection associated with catheters

substitution of antibiotic-containing lubricant for plain lubricant. The results of these studies are conflicting, but the consensus of opinion seems to be that they are valueless.

As for systemic antimicrobial agents, there is little controversy about the necessity to treat established urinary tract infection prior to and during operations, lest the operation result in serious bacteraemia. What is not clear is the place of prophylactic antimicrobial agents in patients without urinary tract infection who undergo urological operations. Chodak and Plaut evaluated 64 reports on the subject and rejected all but 13 on the grounds that the design and conduct of the studies were unsatisfactory.[2] These authors concluded that 'Support for the use of prophylactic antibiotics [in urological surgery] is lacking'.

One of the problems associated with the prophylaxis of infection after prostatectomy is that the prostate itself may be infected even if the urine is not. My practice, therefore, is to give a single intravenous dose of antibiotic effective against Gram-negative aerobes at induction of anaesthesia, just as in all other potentially contaminated abdominal operations. Continuation of prophylaxis for the total duration of catheterization is contra-indicated because it allows the acquisition of resistant strains of microorganisms.

Intermittent or continuous irrigation of the catheterized bladder with antimicrobial solutions is theoretically attractive, and in one study nitrofurantoin irrigation completely abolished catheter-associated urinary infection after transurethral prostatectomy.[3]

Workers in Leiden conducted a random control clinical trial in orthopaedic patients requiring catheterization.[4] Eight of 29 control patients (28 per cent) who had intermittent catheterization developed bacteriuria, compared with one of 28 patients (4 per cent) in whom the bladder was intermittently emptied and then irrigated with 50 ml of 2 per cent povidone iodine solution before withdrawing the catheter.

Intravenous cannulae

Infection is such a common complication of cannulation of peripheral veins that many surgeons insist that the site of intravenous infusion shall be changed every other day. Tully and his colleagues reported lower rates of infection when infusions were given through steel needles than when they were given through plastic cannulae,[5] but that this was probably the result of the shorter life of a needle infusion. When plastic cannulae were left in place for less than 72 hours, the rate of infection did not differ significantly from that associated with steel needles.

Of greater significance in causing serious sepsis is infection of central venous cannulae. These are usually inserted by subclavian vein stab and may be required to remain in use either for monitoring central venous and pulmonary wedge pressures, or for parenteral nutrition, for several weeks. Exogenous bacterial contamination is common, the rate depending partly on the diligence with which it is sought. In a multi-centre study of over 10 000 patients the incidence of clinically important bacteraemia associated with central venous cannulae was reported to be 5.9 per cent.[6]

Technical modifications such as subcutaneous tunnelling of the cannula, and the use of the Hickman cannula incorporating a Dacron cuff, reduce the infection rate. Keohane and his colleagues defined infection as growth of organisms from the tip of the cannula after removal and, in a random control clinical trial, such growth was revealed in 13 of 47 (28 per cent) untunnelled, compared with 6 of 52 (12 per cent) tunnelled, cannulae.[7] The organisms cultured were *Staphylococcus aureus* (9), *Staph. epidermidis* (7), coliforms (3), *Candida albicans* (2) and beta-haemolytic streptococci (i).

The overwhelming importance of meticulous aseptic care of the cannula/ skin interface and of the cannula/reservoir connection is shown in Keohane's study: after 18 months a nutrition nurse joined the team and the rate of cannula tip infection fell to 4 per cent overall and there was no longer any difference between tunnelled and untunnelled cannulae. In Irving's unit, in which total parenteral nutrition is suspended during the day and restarted every night, the rules of asepsis are applied so strictly that no infection has arisen as a result of central venous cannulation in 3 years.[8]

Peritoneal dialysis catheters

As an alternative to haemodialysis in patients with renal failure, peritoneal dialysis is effective and, in the short term, safe. The extension of the technique to long-term treatment of irreversible renal failure by Popovich in 1976 resulted in a high incidence of peritonitis, most often caused by *Staph. epidermidis*. Oreopoulos and his colleagues improved the results by using plastic rather than glass reservoirs for fluid, and demanding that the catheter/ reservoir connection be soaked in povidone iodine solution for 5 minutes at each change of bag.[9] Clark, working in Hong Kong with patients of whom 29 per cent were illiterate, succeeded in eliminating peritonitis in the last 11.5 patient years by several modifications of technique, the most important being the insistence of a timed sterilization by alcoholic chlorhexidine of the catheter/reservoir connection at each change.[10]

Bronchial and pancreatico-biliary catheters

Bacterial contamination of the lower airways by bronchial catheters in patients in intensive care units is common and, in seriously-ill immuno-compromised patients, may lead on to pneumonia (see Chapter 30).

Less common, but equally dangerous, is contamination of bile and pancreatic ducts during endoscopic retrograde cholangio-pancreatography which, in the presence of obstruction, is likely to result in serious infection. The sterilization of endoscopes is difficult, and in many units takes place only after the endoscope has been used. Ridgway and his colleagues contaminated Fujinon OX52 endoscopes with *Pseudomonas aeruginosa* and studied its elimination in a Pauldrach Endocleaner.[11] Twenty minutes of exposure to activated glutaraldehyde resulted in a 99.999 per cent reduction in the number of organisms recovered but, after overnight storage, the endoscopes were found once again to be heavily contaminated. Even if the endoscope, including its air and biopsy/irrigation channel, has been adequately disinfected, there is still the possibility of exogenous or endogenous bacterial contamination of the catheter. For this reason most endoscopists administer a single intravenous dose of a broad-spectrum antibiotic before endoscopic cholangio-pancreatography.

Infections associated with totally implanted devices

The proliferation of these devices within the past 20 years has resulted in improvement in the quality of life for numerous patients, but infection remains a serious problem not only when the device has one end in the potentially-contaminated peritoneal cavity, but even when it is entirely within sterile tissues. Infection of ventriculo-peritoneal and peritoneo-venous shunts can be caused by exogenous skin bacteria or by endogenous intestinal bacteria, whereas infection of cardiac pacemakers and other totally implanted devices for vascular access is nearly always by *Staph. epidermidis* or *Staph. aureus*.[12] The prevention of these infections follows the principles which I have discussed in relation to other operations involving prosthetic implants. Cardiac pacemakers should be inserted only in plenum-ventilated or laminar flow-ventilated operating theatres, meticulous asepsis should be practised, and patients should be given a single dose of an anti-staphylococcal antibiotic before the operation. The antibiotic usually chosen is flucloxacillin, but many strains of *Staph. epidermidis* are resistant, and if the rate of pacemaker infection rises above 1 per cent, the prophylactic antibiotic should be changed to vancomycin.[13]

Conclusions

Indwelling catheters and cannulae which emerge from the skin are at risk of exogenous ward-acquired infection, whereas infections caused by those which are either introduced briefly and then withdrawn (such as endoscopic catheters in the biliary and pancreatic ducts) or are totally implanted, are acquired in the operating theatre. In both cases prophylaxis is primarily by strict observance of asepsis but, in the latter, single-dose pre-operative antibiotic prophylaxis should be added.

References

1. Blenkharn JJ. Prevention of bacteriuria during urinary catheterization of patients in an intensive care unit: evaluation of the 'Ureofix 500' closed drainage system. *J Hosp Infect* 1985; **6**:187–193.
2. Chodak GW, Plaut ME. Systemic antibiotics for prophylaxis in urological surgery: a critical review. *J Urol* 1979; **121**:659–99.
3. Mathew AD, Gonzalez R, Jeffords R, Pinto MH. Prevention of bacteriuria after transurethral prostatectomy with nitrofurantoin macrocrystals. *J Urol* 1978; **120**:442–43.
4. van den Broek PJ, Daha TJ, Mouton RP. Bladder irrigation with povidone iodine in prevention of urinary tract infections associated with intermittent urethral catheterization. *Lancet* 1985; **1**:563–65.
5. Tully JL, Friedland GH, Goldmann DA. Complications of intravenous therapy with steel needles and small-bore teflon catheters. *Am J Med* 1981; **70**:702–706.
6. European Working Party on Control of Hospital Infections. Bacteraemia in surgical patients with intravenous devices: a European multicentre incidence study. *J Hosp Infect* 1983; **4**:338–49.

7. Keohane PP, Attrill H, Northover J, Jones BMJ, Crabb A, Frost P, Silk DBA. Effect of catheter tunnelling and a nutrition nurse on catheter sepsis during parenteral nutrition. A controlled trial. *Lancet* 1983; **ii**:1388–90.

8. Irving M, White R, Tresadern J. Three years' experience with an intestinal failure unit. *Ann Roy Coll Surg Eng* 1985; **67**:1–5.

9. Oreopoulos DG, Robson M, Izatt S, Clayton S, de Veber GA. A simple and safe technique for continuous ambulatory peritoneal dialysis (CAPD). *Trans Am Soc Artif Inter Organs* 1978; **24**:484–89.

10. Clark RD. Peritonitis prevented in continuous ambulatory peritoneal dialysis using the Hong Kong connection. *Brit Med J* 1984; **288**:353–56.

11. Felmingham D, Mowles J, Thomas K, Ridgway GL. Disinfection of gastro-intestinal endoscopes: an evaluation of the Pauldrach Endocleaner and various chemical agents. *J Hosp Infect* 1985; **6**:379–88.

12. Anonymous. Preventing pacemaker infections. *Lancet* 1986; **i**:537–38.

13. Archer GL, Armstrong BC. Alteration in staphylococcal flora in cardiac surgery patients receiving antibiotic prophylaxis. *J Infect Dis* 1983; **147**:642–49.

33

Endogenous ward-acquired infections

Postoperative infections may be caused by a continuation of the infective process which necessitated the operation, by the invasion of bacteria which contaminated the tissues during the operation, by bacteria introduced into the tissues in the recovery period from sources outside the patient or, finally, by bacteria released into the tissues from within the patient's body during the postoperative period. It is with the last of these that I am concerned in this chapter.

Aspiration pneumonia

After major abdominal operations infective intestinal contents can often be identified in the pharynx and, in patients whose ability to cough has been reduced by the presence of an upper abdominal incision, these contents may be aspirated into the lungs where they invade the tissues and cause pneumonia. I discussed the dangerous condition, adult respiratory distress syndrome, in Chapter 7.

Intestinal gangrene

A rare terminal event in seriously ill patients is intestinal gangrene without evidence of arterial or venous occlusion. The condition is usually not discovered until autopsy, and the pathogenesis is obscure. The role of clostridial invasion of the intestinal wall, the defensive capacity of which has been reduced by hypovolaemic or septic shock, is conjectural.

Anastomotic dehiscence

This is the most common cause of serious endogenous postoperatively-acquired sepsis. The healing of an internal anastomosis or suture line in a hollow viscus depends on the balance between collagen lysis and collagen synthesis. For the first week the integrity of the anastomosis is ensured by the sutures or staples which were used to join the tubes together; the gaps between the sutures are sealed by fibrin, which is gradually replaced by the ingrowth of fibroblasts. These cells lay down collagen which is weak but matures into strong bundles arranged along the lines of stress.

The pathogenesis of anastomotic dehiscence is the same as of dehiscence of the abdominal wall after laparotomy. Failure is the result of one of three factors: sutures break, knots slip and tissues tear.[1] Tearing of sutures out of visceral walls is by far the most frequent cause of anastomotic failure, the incidence of which is closely related to the technical skill of the surgeon.[2]

Sutures break

The choice of suture material for internal anastomoses is determined more by tradition and experience than by objective assessment. In biliary and urinary operations the inadvisability of non-absorbable sutures has been conclusively shown: they can form the focus of stone formation. In these organs, therefore, the choice is between natural (catgut) or synthetic (polyglycolic acid, polyglactan, polydioxanone) absorbable sutures. My preference is for monofilament polydioxanone for biliary and pancreatic anastomoses, and catgut in the urinary system; the rate of hydrolytic disintegration of polyglycolic acid is enhanced by contact with urine.[3] For gastro-duodenal suture lines I use an inner (haemostatic) layer of continuous catgut and an outer layer of either catgut or braided polyester, depending on my estimate of the time it will take for the healing process to be far enough advanced not to need the integrity of the sutures.

For intestinal anastomoses, and particularly for those involving the oeso-phagus and the rectum, I choose sutures the strength of which will persist until healing is far advanced; there does not appear to be anything to recommend any particular material.

Knots slip

This is a rare cause of anastomotic failure. Braided materials knot more securely than monofilament materials, but a knot that comes untied is a knot badly made.

Tissues tear

The strongest suture most securely tied will be of no avail if the tissues joined by that suture disintegrate and allow the suture to tear out. Why should the tissue disintegrate? I suggest that there are several possible causes; these can be broadly classified as either mechanical or microbiological, but the most potent is bacterial invasion at the site of anastomosis.

- The sutures were inserted too near the cut edges. It is generally accepted that a 5 mm 'bite' of tissue on each side is desirable, and we showed in a controlled clinical trial of colonic anastomoses that 10 mm bites were no more secure than 5 mm bites.[4]
- The sutures did not include the strong submucosal layer of intestine. The importance of this layer was shown by Halsted;[5] anastomoses in which the sutures do not embrace the submucosa can fail.
- There was so much tension on the anastomosis that purely mechanical forces tore the sutures out of the bowel. The avoidance of tension is a fundamental rule in making any internal anastomosis and, in performing an anastomosis to the rectum, the peritoneal attachments of the splenic flexure must be divided and the transverse colon displaced downwards.

- The blood supply to one end of the intestine was so poor that the tissue embraced by the sutures disintegrated from necrosis. In elective intestinal resections this is rare, surgeons being careful to ensure that both ends of the bowel bleed freely. It is a more common complication of emergency resection of small intestine which is gangrenous as a result of strangulation or arterial occlusion. In these cases one or both ends of the remaining intestine may be ischaemic and, after anastomosis, become completely gangrenous. The possibility of this tragedy should be borne in mind, and either the intestinal ends exteriorized to be anastomosed later, or the abdomen re-opened the following day with a view to further resection if necessary.
- The blood supply, although apparently adequate at the time of operation, was insufficient to enable an efficient inflammatory reaction to take place. In this case bacterial action itself can result in necrosis of the tissues embraced by the sutures.
- Even in well-vascularized bowel, the bacterial contamination at the site of anastomosis was great enough to overcome the local resistance and cause necrosis. The importance both of a clean intestine and of adequate tissue concentrations of appropriate antibiotics cannot be overstressed.
- The inflammatory reaction was proceeding satisfactorily and new collagen was being laid down, but an abscess contiguous to the anastomosis broke through the suture line. This is the traditional explanation of the failure of anastomoses to the subperitoneal rectum or anal canal and the theoretical justification for external drainage of the presacral space. These drains, the function of which is to evacuate blood and serum which – if left undisturbed – might nourish bacteria, should be removed after no more than 48 hours lest the drains themselves cause pressure necrosis at the anastomosis.

Results of anastomotic dehiscence

A small anastomotic defect may be so adequately contained by surrounding tissues that it causes no clinical problems and may be detected only by contrast X-ray studies. On the other hand, it may result in a local abscess or faecal fistula. If the defect is large and uncontained, the result is general peritonitis, and all the consequences of sepsis (see Chapter 7).

The diagnosis of anastomotic dehiscence

Subclinical leaks

A complete and honest audit requires recognition of small leaks as well as those which cause clinical illness. In patients with an anastomosis to the rectum or anal canal it is my practice to request a gentle water-soluble X-ray contrast enema on about the tenth postoperative day in order to discover subclinical leaks. This technique was introduced by Goligher in 1970[6] and revealed a much higher rate of dehiscence than had previously been suspected.

General peritonitis

Rapid deterioration in a patient's condition with signs of septic shock a few days after an internal anastomosis should always be provisionally attributed to uncontained anastomotic dehiscence rather than to any other cause. Abdominal examination seldom shows the board-like rigidity found in patients with visceral perforations, and the differentiation from cardiogenic shock may be difficult. Peritoneal lavage or X-ray contrast studies may be indicated, but the most important pointer is a high index of suspicion.

Faecal fistula

The discharge of intestinal contents through a drain or through the wound is a clear indication of anastomotic failure. It is sometimes difficult at first to distinguish the fluid from pus or peritoneal fluid, but the distinction usually becomes clear within a day or two.

Abscess

Intra-abdominal abscesses may result from community-acquired infections, in particular those which follow perforation of a hollow viscus. They may, however, develop as a result of a well-contained leak from an internal suture line. The common sites are pelvic, paracolic and central abdominal; subphrenic and subhepatic abscesses are relatively rare. The diagnosis of an intra-abdominal abscess depends initially on clinical observations. The body temperature is raised and blood count shows a polymorphonuclear leucocytosis; the patient is ill. A mass may be felt in the abdomen or on rectal examination, and a pleural effusion is a constant accompaniment of a subphrenic abscess. For the accurate localization of an intra-abdominal abscess, however, three additional diagnostic measures are available.

Ultrasound scan

In the hands of an expert the diagnosis of loculated fluid anywhere in the abdomen is relatively easy, unless bowel gas obscures the lesion. The success of the examination is, however, dependent on the skill of the operator. The method has several advantages, including non-invasiveness, cheapness and availability at the bedside.

Computerized tomography

This is an equally accurate method of diagnosis and is less dependent on skill. Contrast enhancement of X-ray opacity of hollow or solid organs is often a help in precise localization of an abscess.

Isotope scan

Mixed leucocytes (the buffy coat of spun plasma) can be labelled with radio-active isotopes of chromium, phosphorus,[7] technetium,[8] gallium[9] or indium.[10] These labelled cells accumulate not only in the liver, spleen and bone marrow, but also in abscesses where they can be imaged by gamma camera. The most successful isotope clinically appears to be [111]indium, but the detection of abscesses around the liver and spleen depends on subtracting the images of those organs obtained by a technetium-colloid scan. The technique of *in vitro* labelling of leucocytes is complicated and expensive, and perhaps the future lies in the discovery of an isotope compound which can be injected intravenously and will selectively accumulate within abscesses.

Treatment of anastomotic dehiscence

Minor defects with no clinical symptoms require no immediate treatment, but the extramural fibrosis associated with the eventual healing may result in a stricture which requires dilatation or even, occasionally, resection. Faecal fistulae nearly always resolve with conservative treatment including, in the case of a high-output fistula, parenteral nutrition.

Well-localized abscesses may need to be drained, and percutaneous drainage under ultrasound control – or the site having been determined by computerized tomography – is preferable to laparotomy. There are exceptions: the method is unsuitable when the pus is highly viscous, when the abscess is multilocular or when it is associated with extensive tissue necrosis, as is the case with a pancreatic abscess. There is, however, no longer any indication for exploratory laparotomy: the site and extent of an abscess must be precisely known before operation.

When the anastomotic breakdown is massive and causes general peritonitis and sepsis, the treatment is primarily surgical, accompanied by parenteral administration of antimicrobial agents active against both aerobic and anaerobic bacteria. The surgical choices are either diversion of the contents of the viscus by proximal exteriorization, exteriorization of the anastomosis if that is technically feasible, or taking down the anastomosis and exteriorizing the proximal component. A difficult problem arises when there has been a massive dehiscence of an oesophago-intestinal, gastro-intestinal or duodenal suture line. Conservative treatment merely by drainage of an abscess is unlikely to save these patients, and some method of defunctioning the leaking anastomosis should be used. This may involve cervical oesophagostomy or Billroth II gastrectomy. The mortality rate is high, in the region of 70 per cent in some series. No attempt should be made to repair an anastomotic defect either by suture or by re-resection and anastomosis: in the presence of sepsis a new suture line will usually fail.

Conclusion

The main cause of endogenous postoperatively-acquired infection is failure of an internal suture line in a hollow viscus. Anastomotic dehiscences are preventable by paying attention to all the technical rules; anastomotic dehiscences may, however, result in minimal clinical symptoms, or they may cause localized abscesses. Massive breakdown of an anastomosis results in serious peritonitis and sepsis, and requires antibiotics and resuscitation, followed by operation to exteriorize the anastomosis.

References

1. Leaper DJ, Pollock AV, Evans M. Abdominal wound closure: a trial of nylon, polyglycolic acid and steel sutures. *Brit J Surg* 1977; **64**:603–606.
2. Fielding LP, Stewart-Brown S, Blesovsky L, Kearney G. Anastomotic integrity after operations for large-bowel cancer: a multicentre study. *Brit Med J* 1980; **2**:411–14.
3. Holbrook MC. The breakdown of PGA in human urine. *Brit J Surg* 1978; **65**: 361.
4. Greenall MJ, Evans M, Pollock AV. Influence of depth of suture bite on integrity of single-layer large-bowel anastomoses. *J Roy Soc Med* 1979; **72**:351–56.
5. Halsted WS. Circular suture of the intestine – an experimental study. *Am J Med Sci* 1887; **94**:436–61.
6. Goligher JC, Graham NG, de Dombal FT. Anastomotic dehiscence after anterior resection of rectum and sigmoid. *Brit J Surg* 1970; **57**:109–18.
7. Dresch C, Najean V, Beauchet J. *In vitro* 51-Cr and 32-P-DFP labeling of granulocytes in man. *J Nuclear Med* 1971; **12**:774–85.
8. Anderson, BR, English D, Akalin HE, Henderson W. Inflammatory lesions localized with technetium Tc 99m-labeled leukocytes. *Arch Intern Med 1975;* **135**:1067–71.
9. Deysine M, Robinson, R, Rafkin H, Teicher I, Silver L, Aufses H Jr. Clinical infections detected by 67-Ga scanning. *Ann Surg* 1974; **180**:897–901.
10. Thakur ML, Coleman RE, Mayhall CG, Welch MJ Jr. Preparation and evaluation of 111-In-labeled leukocyctes as an abscess imaging agent in dogs. *Radiology* 1976; **119**:731–32.

34

Infections in immunocompromised patients

Immunity to infection depends first and foremost on the integrity of skin and mucosa and the ability of mucosal surfaces to resist microbial attachment by ciliary action or the formation of a mucous barrier. Secondly, it depends on the efficient functioning of all components of the immune system (see Chapter 4).

Primary immune defects

Congenital defects in mucosal integrity, for example those found in cystic fibrosis, and of humoral and cellular components of the immune system, are of great interest to immunologists and of concern to paediatricians. These patients seldom present with surgical infections, and I do not propose considering them further.

Secondary immune defects

The immune system may be compromised by starvation, disease, drugs and operations. In all cases infection results only after a failure of the integument to prevent entry of microorganisms. The skin may be breached by intravenous cannulae, the bronchial mucosa by endotracheal tubes or by aspiration of gastric acid, and the intestinal or vesical mucosa by radiotherapy or cytotoxic drugs. Adherence to, and invasion of, mucosal surfaces by microorganisms are normally prevented by the 'washing' effect of cilia, tears, intestinal secretions and urine; disturbances of these mechanisms predispose to infection.

Causes of immune deficiency

Immune defects as a result of malnutrition

Starving people in the Third World suffer and die from all manner of viral, bacterial and protozoal infections. Frank starvation is uncommon in Western countries, but it has been assumed that lesser degrees of malnutrition may predispose to septic complications after operations. Research has concentrated on two questions: how do we define the degrees of malnutrition, and do attempts to correct malnutrition help our patients?

Definition of malnutrition

Clinical judgement is reasonably reliable, but it is subject to bias and observer variability; most workers, therefore, prefer objective assessments. The Prognostic Nutritional Index is comprised of four measurements – serum levels of albumin and transferrin, triceps skin-fold thickness and the degree of cell-mediated immune competence revealed by delayed hypersensitivity skin tests.[1] Linn devised a more complete scoring system based on four categories – clinical history, physical examination, anthropometric measurements and laboratory tests.[2] This he called the Protein Energy Malnutrition Scale.

Meakins and his colleagues concentrated on the results of delayed hypersensitivity skin tests to five antigens (candida, mumps, purified protein derivative of old tuberculin, trichophyton and streptokinase/streptodornase).[3] They tested patients before operation and 1 week later. The overall mortality rate was 20.6 per cent and this correlated closely with the degree of anergy revealed by skin tests. When patients reacted normally to two or more antigens before and after operation, 1 out of 83 died; when the pre-operative tests showed anergy or relative anergy (reaction to none or one antigen) but the postoperative test was normal, 4 out of 94 died; when, however, the test either remained or became abnormal, 46 out of 59 died. This experience was not confirmed by workers in Manchester[4] or in my own unit.[5] A group of workers in Toronto compared clinical judgement with the results of a battery of anthropometric, biochemical and delayed hypersensitivity skin tests in assessing 48 surgical patients.[6] They classified them into three categories: *normal* (25 patients who stayed in hospital an average of 18.4 days and of whom 4 suffered postoperative infections), *mildly malnourished* (7 patients, who stayed in hospital an average of 25.4 days and of whom 3 suffered postoperative infections) and *severely malnourished* (16 patients, who stayed in hospital an average of 48.6 days and of whom 11 suffered postoperative infections). They concluded that 'carefully performed history taking and physical examination are sufficient for nutritional assessment'.

Does correction of malnutrition help surgical patients?

In Western countries malnutrition is almost always caused by disease, and there is no evidence that pre-operative enteral or parenteral hyperalimentation has any effect on the outcome of an operation for the relief of that disease.[7] On the contrary, correction of some deficiencies – notably of iron – may have quite the reverse effect. The Murrays studied Somali nomads in the Ogaden and found iron deficiency in a high proportion.[8] As they had only a limited supply of ferrous sulphate tablets, they gave these to about half their patients, and aluminium hydroxide tablets to the remainder. Twenty-seven of the 71 patients whose iron deficiency was corrected suffered 36 episodes of infection, including recrudescences of malaria, brucellosis and tuberculosis. Only 5 of the 66 nomads given placebo tablets suffered infections.

On the other hand, the place of total parenteral nutrition in the supplementary treatment of spontaneous or postoperative high intestinal fistulae and of complicated intra-abdominal sepsis is well-established.

Specific nutritional deficiencies

In animals deficiencies of zinc, copper, magnesium and selenium have been shown to interfere with the efficient functioning of the immune system. Such mineral deficiencies are, however, rare in clinical practice and attempts to improve the response to trauma and infection by administration of any of these minerals have not shown convincing benefits.

The role of vitamin deficiencies in reducing the host response to infections is equally controversial, except in the case of frank scurvy, but scurvy without protein-calorie malnutrition and deficiencies of other vitamins is rare. Subclinical scurvy shown by failure to excrete a large proportion of injected ascorbic acid is probably of no significance.

Immune defects as a result of diseases

Uncontrolled diabetes, hepatic and renal failure and disseminated cancer all interfere with aspects of the immune system and increase the liability of the patient to serious infections. There is an increased risk of postoperative wound infections in the obese and the aged. In a personal series of 939 operations I found a higher incidence of wound infection in fat young people than in those people whose thickness of subcutaneous fat at the site of incision was less than 2.5 cm.[9] This difference was not apparent in patients over the age of 65 years, the rate of total wound infection – major and minor – depended not on age, but on the extent of operative bacterial contamination. When a wound became infected in an old person, however, the infection was significantly more likely to be major. These findings are probably related to the relative avascularity of both obese and aged tissues.

Acute leukaemias and disseminated lymphomas or carcinomas produce immune defects by replacing bone marrow and throttling the production of immunologically active cells. Patients with active Crohn's disease usually show no hypersensitivity response to intradermally-injected antigens: this reflects a depression of cell-mediated immunity and may account for some of the infections which complicate operations in these patients.

Certain viral diseases – measles is the best-documented example – so depress the host's ability to fight infections that they are important causes of death from complicating bacterial infections in children in developing countries.

Acquired immune deficiency syndrome (AIDS)

This infection by the human immunodeficiency virus (HIV) affects mainly promiscuous homosexual men and the incidence appears to be increasing exponentially. It is detected by the presence of serum antibodies to the virus and most cases are asymptomatic or suffer a self-limiting glandular fever-like illness with generalized lymphadenopathy. The full-blown picture of AIDS includes severe immunosuppression which allows opportunistic infections, the commonest being by *Pneumocystis carinii*. Approximately 25 per cent of all patients with AIDS will develop Kaposi's sarcoma. From the surgical point of view the dangers of operating on a patient with AIDS are two fold: postoperative infections in the patient are common, and a needle-stick injury to the surgeon or other member of the operating team may inoculate the virus infection in them.

Immune defects caused by drugs

Immune suppression is the goal of drug treatment after organ transplantation, whereas it is an unwanted side-effect of treatment in many other conditions. Steroids in high doses or for prolonged periods affect all aspects of cellular, humoral and neutrophil defences. The antimetabolites azathioprine and cyclosporin act specifically on lymphocytes, depressing immunoglobulin production by B-cells and preventing the acquisition of receptors for interleukin-1 and -2 and the release of lymphokines which stimulate the production of cytotoxic T-cells. The cytotoxic drugs which are used to control the growth of some cancers affect all the cells of the immune system, and careful monitoring of the peripheral white blood cells is necessary to forestall gross leucopenia. Similar defects may complicate radiotherapy.

Immune defects as a result of trauma

Many aspects of the immune system are depressed by trauma, and the greater the trauma the more the suppression.

Lymphocytes and cell-mediated immunity

The advent of monoclonal antibodies has allowed the separation of lymphocytes into B-cells and three populations of T-cells:[10] helper/inducer (OKT 4, Leu-3a), suppressor/cytotoxic (OKT-8, Leu-2a) and natural killer cells. When differentially stained with fluorescein-conjugated monoclonal antibodies, the numbers in each population can be estimated by flow cytometry in a fluorescence-activated cell sorter (FACS 420). Following trauma all subsets of T-cells show a reduction,[11] but this is most marked in the OKT-4 cells, resulting in a relative increase in OKT-8 suppressor/cytotoxic cells. This disturbance returns to normal in a few days unless systemic sepsis occurs, in which case the relative preponderance of OKT-8 cells persists and the patient may die.[12]

   The disturbances of T-lymphocyte production are reflected in the anergy when patients are tested by skin hypersensitivity reactions to recall antigens after severe trauma. This is most notable after extensive burns and accounts for the slow rejection of skin allografts in these patients.

Neutrophil function

The normal reaction to trauma is a neutrophil leucocytosis. The increase in neutrophil numbers may not, however, be matched by improvement in their function of bacterial killing. Alexander and his colleagues studied the neutrophil bactericidal index – the proportion of *Staphylococcus aureus* surviving incubation with neutrophils – after severe burns and found the killing function reduced.[13] The degree of reduction correlated with sepsis.

Christou and Meakins studied the adherence to a nylon filter of neutrophils and their chemotaxis into a micropore filter.[14] They found that in anergic patients (judged by failure to respond to intradermal antigens) adherence increased and chemotaxis decreased.

Humoral immunosuppressant activity after major trauma

Several plasma proteins have immunosuppressive activity and estimation, after major operations, of alpha-1-proteinase inhibitor, alpha-2-pregnancy-associated glycoprotein and plasma suppressive activity on stimulated lymphocytes showed increased levels.[11] Alpha-2-macroglobulin paradoxically showed a fall, but this is probably explained by the finding that breakdown of the alpha-2-macroglobulin-protease complex releases another immunosuppressive peptide.[15]

Immune defects as a result of blood transfusion

Recipients of renal allografts are less likely to reject their grafts if they have had blood transfusion.[16] Recurrence of breast[17] and colon[18] cancer is more often encountered in patients who have been transfused in the peri-operative period than in those who have not been transfused. There appears, therefore, to be a specific immunodeficiency state produced by blood transfusion. Whether this defect applies only to cell-mediated immunity and whether it is an important determinant of surgical bacterial infections is at present conjectural.

Prophylaxis and treatment of infections in patients with secondary immune defects

I will consider four aspects of the care of immunosuppressed patients: the prevention of exogenous infections, the prevention of endogenous infections, the correction of immune defects and the treatment of infections in immunocompromised patients.

Prevention of exogenous infections

All the rules which I have discussed in relation to hospital-acquired infections must be applied even more strictly when dealing with immunocompromised patients. Any break in the integument of skin or mucosa may allow the invasion of bacteria, and attendants must be warned not to risk such breaks. This applies not only to the prevention of pressure necrosis of the skin, but also to the avoidance of rectal examinations, sigmoidoscopy, urethral catheterization, endotracheal intubation and indwelling venous cannulae. It may be impossible to avoid some of these invasive measures but, if they are absolutely necessary, the attendants should be aware of the increased risks of infection associated with them and the rules of asepsis should be observed even more rigorously than in patients with an intact immune system. *Pseudomonas aeruginosa* is a common cause of septicaemia in severely immunocompromised patients and can contaminate any aqueous solution.[19] Special attention to sterilization and asepsis is necessary in intensive care units.

Protective isolation

For patients with profound depression of immune capability, particularly those whose cytotoxic treatment has reduced the blood neutrophil count to less then $1.0 \times 10^9/dl$, some form of protective isolation is needed. There are serious logistic and psychological problems inherent in the most extreme forms of isolation, and it is common practice to nurse such patients in rooms with positive-pressure ventilation and to enforce hand disinfection on the few people who are allowed to enter that room. Hands are far more important than noses or clothing in the spread of exogenous organisms. Provided the hands are socially clean, all that is needed is to apply an alcoholic solution of chlorhexidine and allow it to dry on the skin. Sterile gloves must be worn when any invasive treatment is carried out.

Prevention of endogenous infections

It is impossible to sterilize a patient's skin and gastro-intestinal tract, but we can achieve partial decontamination. The patient should be washed with chlorhexidine detergent instead of soap; this undoubtedly reduces the skin burden of *Staph. epidermidis*, but probably has little effect on the incidence of infection. Gut decontamination is more controversial. On the one hand it is perfectly easy to reduce the number of faecal organisms by any of a large number of antibacterial substances but, on the other hand, disturbance of the normal bacterial ecology in the colon usually allows the overgrowth of resistant strains of bacteria and fungi. Furthermore, absorption of orally-administered antibacterials may encourage the emergence of resistant micro-organisms in the lungs and blood stream. Nevertheless, clinical trials have shown a reduction in the number of bacteraemic episodes in patients receiving oral aminoglycosides, erythromycin base, trimethoprim, colistin, polymyxin B, nalidixic acid, metronidazole and vancomycin. In the treatment of patients with severe neutropenia, a combination of two or more of these drugs is indicated.[20]

Experience in Groningen[21] and in Glasgow (S. Alcock, personal communication) has shown the value of a combination of pharyngeal and gastric administration of tobramycin, polymyxin and amphotericin in controlling nosocomial infections in intensive care units. Patients were given a cephalosporin systemically for 4 days until gut decontamination was achieved. In Groningen this regimen reduced the rate of nosocomial infections to 16 per cent in patients who had suffered severe trauma and were intubated and mechanically ventilated. This contrasted with an infection rate of 81 per cent in historical controls given no prophylactic antibiotics.

Correction of immune defects

The advent of antibiotics 40 years ago temporarily eclipsed work on immunoregulators, but the growing problems of bacterial resistance have once again focused attention on measures to correct immune defects. In 1945 Freund produced an antigen by extraction from cultures of *Mycobacterium tuberculosis* which he called Complete Adjuvant.[22] This proved too toxic for clinical use, but a refined extract, muramyl dipeptide, shows promise in experimental animals.[23]

Levamisole, originally introduced and still extensively used in veterinary practice as an anthelmintic, has been shown to have immune restorative properties. Its place in clinical practice has not been established, and work in my unit failed to show benefit from peri-operative administration of the drug.[24]

Vaccination of immunocompromised patients can fail if the production of immunoglobulins is inefficient and, in those who are severely compromised, vaccination may actually increase the risks. Passive immunization by hyper-immune human globulin may have a role in the prevention of infections by cytomegalovirus and possibly *Ps. aeruginosa*, and antiserum to the core lipopolysaccharide of J5 *Escherichia coli* may prevent endotoxic shock but probably not infection.[25]

Theoretically, it is logical to transfuse neutrophils in patients with severe leucopenia. There are, however, two drawbacks: in the first place the neutrophils have a life of only a few hours and, secondly, they may cause the production of antibodies to the host's own neutrophils.

Finally, it is even more essential in immunocompromised patients than in others to ensure that tissue oxygenation is adequate. Blood volume replacement, attention to profound anaemia and the administration of oxygen all play a part.

Treatment of infections in the immunocompromised patient[26]

Many of these infections are polymicrobial and the distinction between colonization and infection can be difficult. Both these aspects militate against accurate and specific antibiotic therapy. Any patient whose immune competence is impaired and who is pyrexial, or shows other signs of infection, should be given broad-spectrum antibiotics, and there is no proof that any of the newer drugs is any better than the combination of gentamicin and mezlocillin. The place of the new quinolone derivatives such as ciprofloxacin remains to be defined.

Before starting antibiotic treatment specimens of blood, urine, sputum and any discharge should be cultured under aerobic and anaerobic conditions, but it is not safe to await the results of the cultures before giving antibiotics. In patients who have had a recent operation, careful search must be made for an infection related to the operation; in the abdomen the most reliable imaging techniques for the presence of an abscess are ultrasound and computerized tomography. Radiographs of the chest may suggest *P. carinii* infection, which should be confirmed by open lung biopsy and treated by co-trimoxazole (trimethoprim/sulphamethoxazole). In patients who have received antibiotics one should always remember the possibility of disseminated fungal infection which requires treatment by nystatin or amphotericin B. Finally, disseminated or locally destructive viral infections, particularly by herpes simplex virus, are common, and the results of acyclovir treatment are generally disappointing.

Summary

Immunity to infection depends initially on integrity of skin and mucosa and the efficiency of functioning of antibacterial mechanisms in the integuments. If microorganisms are permitted access to the tissues, the defences against infection are both humoral and cellular. These defences can be compromised by malnutrition, disease, drugs, trauma and blood transfusions. In the treatment of immunosuppressed patients attention must be paid to the prevention of exogenous and endogenous bacterial contamination, to measures to correct immune defects, and to the energetic and responsible use of antibiotics and the surgical drainage of abscesses.

References

1. Buzby GP, Mullen JL, Matthews DC, Hobbs CL, Rosato EF. Prognostic nutritional index in gastrointestinal surgery. *Am J Surg* 1980; **139**:160–67.
2. Linn BS. A protein energy malnutrition score (PEMS). *Ann Surg* 1984; **200**: 747–52.
3. Meakins JL, Pietsch JB, Christou NV, Maclean LD. Predicting surgical infection before the operation. *World J Surg* 1980; **4**:439–50.
4. Brown R, Bancewicz J, Hamid J, Tillotson G, Ward C, Irving MH. Delayed hypersensitivity skin testing does not influence the management of surgical patients. *Ann Surg* 1982; **196**:672–76.
5. Ausobsky JR, Bean P, Proctor J, Pollock AV. Delayed hypersensitivity testing for the prediction of postoperative complications. *Br J Surg* 1982; **69**:346–48.
6. Baker, JP, Detsky AS, Wesson DE, Wohnan SL, Stewart S, Whitewell J, Langer B, Jeejeebhoy KN. Nutritional assessment. A comparison of clinical judgement and objective measurements. *New Eng J Med* 1982; **306**:969–72.
7. Rennie MJ, Harrison R. Effects of injury, disease and malnutrition on protein metabolism in man. Unanswered questions. *Lancet* 1984; **i**:323–25.
8. Murray MJ, Murray AB, Murray MB, Murray CJ. The adverse effect of iron repletion on the course of certain infections. *Br Med J* 1978; **2**: 1113–15.
9. Pollock AV, Evans M. Surgical wound infection: the influence of age and obesity. *SE Asian J Surg* 1984; **7**:243–47.
10. Kung PC, Goldstein, G, Reinherz EL, Schlossman SF. Monoclonal antibodies defining distinctive human T-cell antigens. *Science* 1979; **206**: 347–49.
11. Lennard TWJ, Shenton BK, Borzotta A, Donnelly PK, White M, Gerrie LM, Proud G, Taylor RMR. The influence of surgical operations on components of the human immune system. *Br J Surg* 1985; **72**:771–76.
12. McIrvine AJ, O'Mahoney JB, Saporoschetz I, Mannick JA. Depressed immune response in burn patients. Use of monoclonal antibodies and functional assays to define the role of suppressor cells. *Ann Surg* 1982; **196**:294–304.
13. Alexander JW, Dionigi R, Stinnett JD. Detection of defects in host defence mechanisms and their repair in the infection-prone patient. In: Burke JF, Hildick Smith GY. (Eds) *The Infection-Prone Hospital Patient*. Boston, Little, Brown & Co., 1978, pp 51–70.
14. Christou NV, Meakins JL. Neutrophil function in anergic surgical patients: neutrophil adherence and chemotaxis. *Ann Surg* 1979; **190**: 557–64.
15. Donnelly PK, Shenton BK, Alomvan AH, Francis DMA, Proud G, Taylor RMR. The role of protease in immunoregulation. *Br J Surg* 1983; **70**:614–22.
16. Proud G, Shenton BK, Smith BM. Blood transfusion and renal transplantation. *Br J Surg* 1979; **66**:678–82.

17. Tartter PI, Burrows L, Papatestas AE, Lesnick G, Aufses AH. Perioperative blood transfusion has prognostic significance for breast cancer. *Surgery* 1985; **97**:225-30.
18. Blumberg N, Agarwal MM, Chuang C. Relation between recurrence of cancer of the colon and blood transfusion. *Br Med J* 1985; **290**: 1037-39.
19. Stephenson JR, Heard SR, Richards MA, Tabaqchali S. Gastrointestinal colonization and septicaemia with *Pseudomonas aeruginosa* due to contaminated thymol mouthwash in immunocompromised patients. *J Hosp Infect* 1985; **6**:369-78.
20. Wade JC, Schimpff SC, Hargadon MT, Fortner CL, Young VM, Wiernik PH. A comparison of trimethoprim-sulfamethoxazole plus nystatin with gentamicin plus nystatin in the prevention of infections in acute leukaemia. *New Eng J Med* 1981; **304**:1057-62.
21. Stoutenbeek CP, van Saene HKF, Miranda DR, Zandstra DF, Binnendijk B. The prevention of superinfection in multiple trauma patients. *J Antimicrob Chemother* 1984; **14 Suppl B**: 203-211.
22. Freund J, Sommer HE, Walter AW. Immunization against malaria: vaccination of ducks with killed parasites incorporated with adjuvants. *Science* 1945; **102**:200-202.
23. Polk HC Jr, Galland RB, Ausobsky JR. Nonspecific enhancement of resistance to bacterial infection. Evidence of an effect supplemental to antibiotics. *Ann Surg* 1982; **196**:436-41.
24. Ausobsky JR, Evans M, Pollock AV. Levamisole and postoperative complications. A controlled clinical trial. *Br J Surg* 1982; **69**:447-48.
25. Baumgartner J-D, Glauser MP, McCutchan JA, Ziegler EJ, van Melle G, Klauber MR, Vogt M, Euehlen E, Luethy R, Chiolero R, Geroulanos S. Prevention of Gram-negative shock and death in surgical patients by antibody to endotoxin core glycolipid. *Lancet* 1985; **ii**:59-63.
26. Marcus RE, Goldman JM. Management of infection in the neutropenic patient. *Br Med J* 1986; **293**:406-408.

Index